MDSAP

Vol.2 of 5 Brazil

For All

(Employees & Employers)

Second Edition:

Online Certification

www.silosa.ca

Jahangir Asadi

Vancouver, BC CANADA

Published by: Top Ten Award International Network Inc.
Vancouver, BC **CANADA**
Email: Info@TopTenAward.net
www.TopTenAward.org

Ordering Information:
Quantity sales. Special discounts are available on quantity purchases by universities, schools, corporations, associations, and others. For details, contact the "Sales Department" at the above mentioned email address.

MDSAP Vol.1-5 (for all employees and employers)/J.Asadi—2nd ed.
ISBN: 978-1-990451-60-7 Vol.1 Australia Hardcover
ISBN: 978-1-990451-61-4 Vol.2 Brazil Hardcover
ISBN: 978-1-990451-62-1 Vol.3 Canada Hardcover
ISBN: 978-1-990451-63-8 Vol.4 Japan Hardcover
ISBN: 978-1-990451-64-5 Vol.5 USA Hardcover

Contents

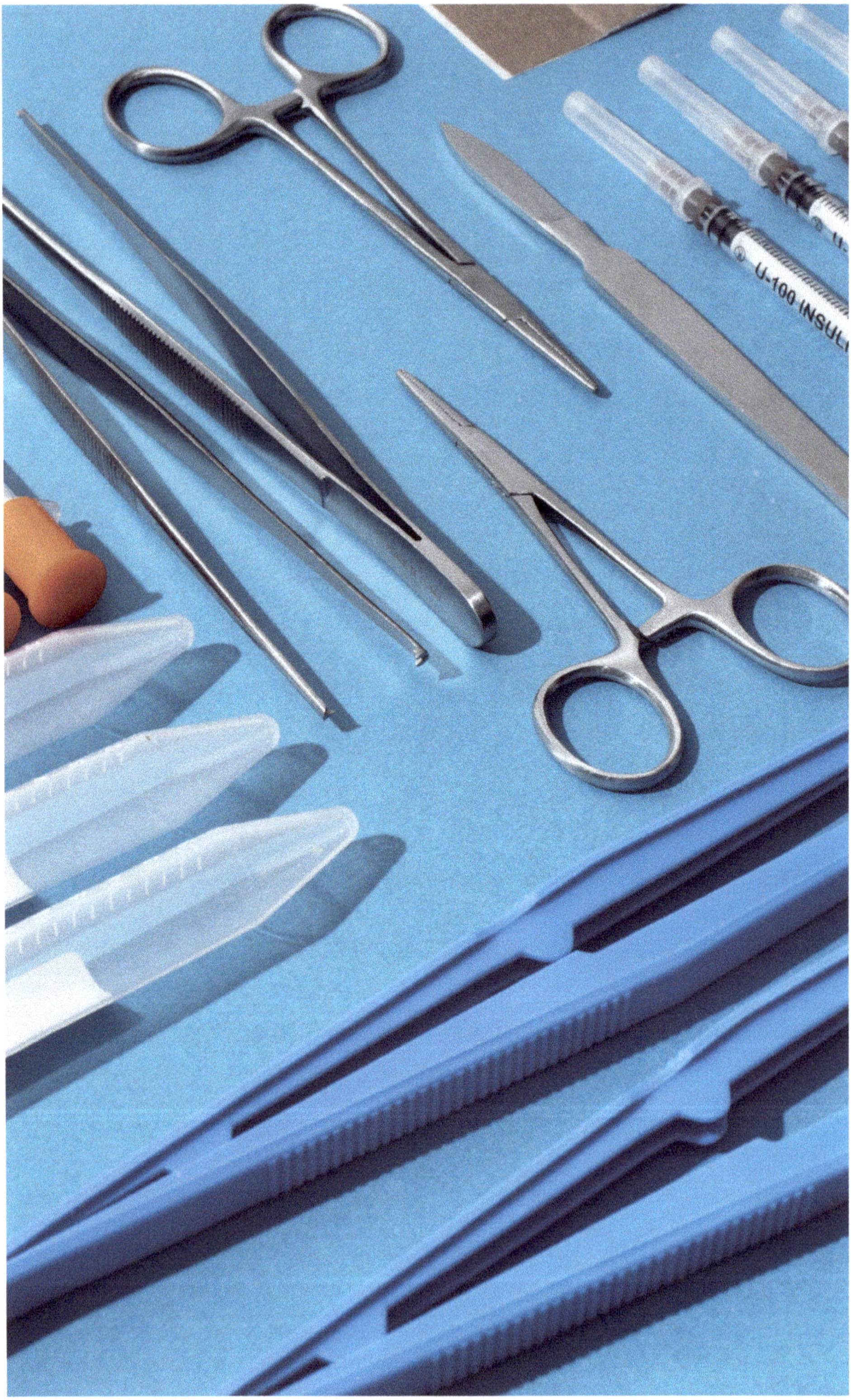
U-100 INSUL

This book is dedicated to my first manager,

Mir Ahmad Sadat,

a Distinguished man of ISIRI, who has been my supporter and has encouraged me greatly and believed genuinely in my ability with honesty and self-confidence.

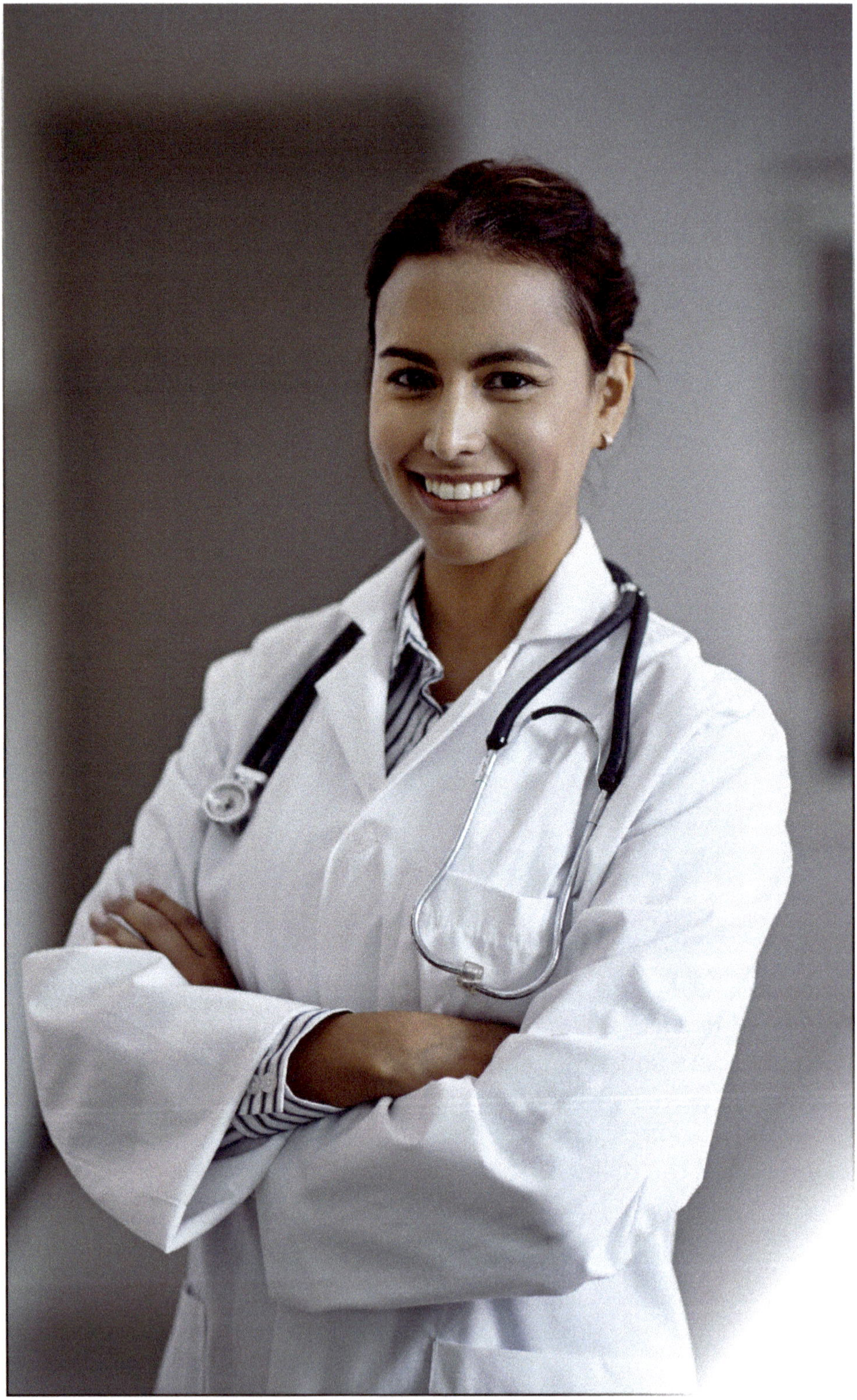

SILOSA Consulting Group (SCG)

Silosa Consulting Group (SCG) was established to provide outstanding consulting services of management system standards to individuals, groups, companies, and organizations all over the globe.
SCG is publishing an "EASY ISO" book series related to International Management System Standards to increase public knowledge in implementing these systems over their organizations.
SCG book publishing services and distribution services are connected to over 39,000 booksellers worldwide, including Apple, Amazon, Barnes & Noble, Indigo, Google Play Books, and many more.
We focus on quality, environmental, food safety and other management system standards.

SCG has enough experiences to help create new and effective programmes in different countries all over the world. For more detail, visit our
website : http://silosa.ca and/or send your enquiery to the following email:

info@silosa.ca

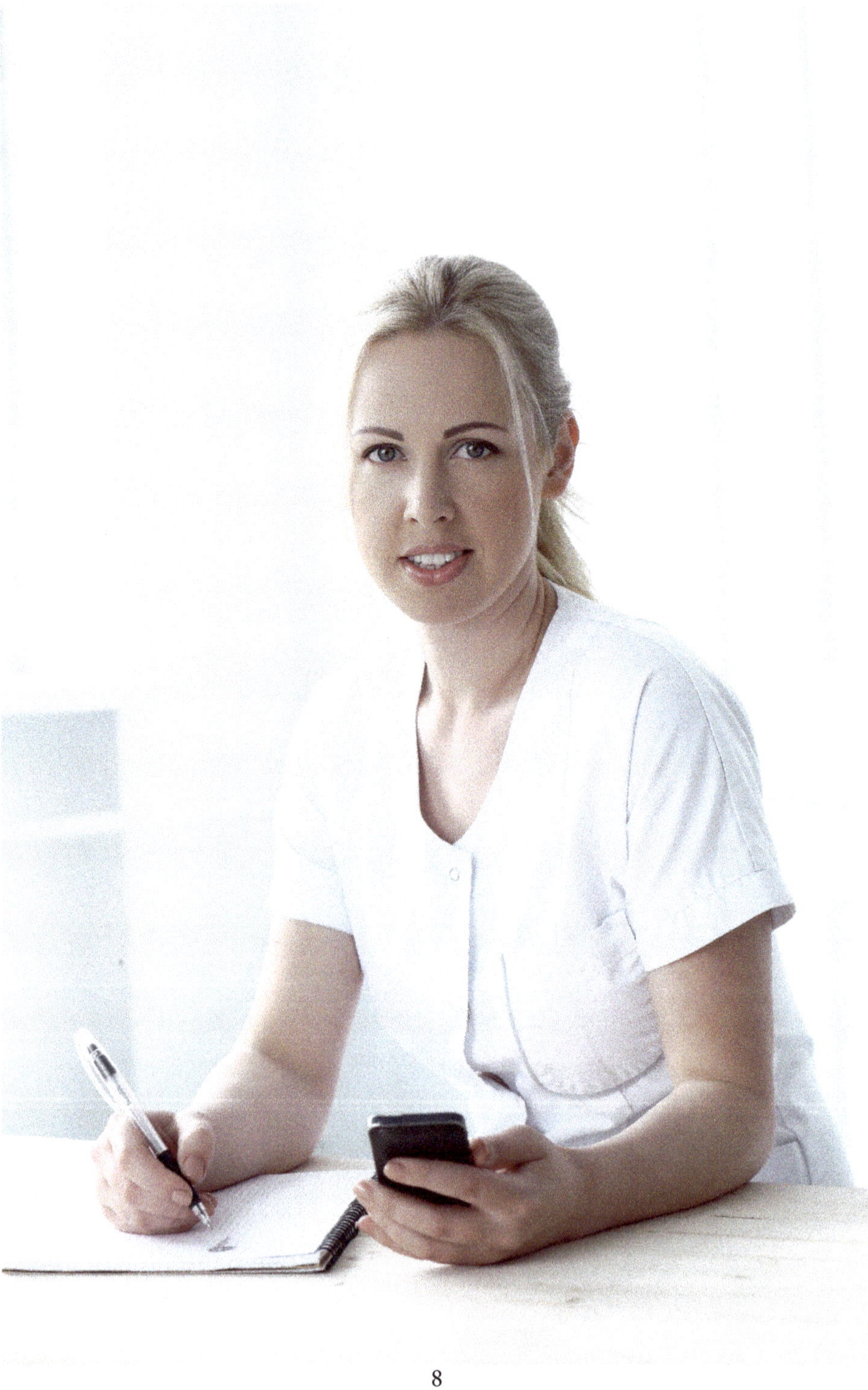

CHAPTER 1

About ISO

The International Organization for Standardization is an independent, non-governmental organization, the members of which are the standards organizations of the 165 member countries. It is the world's largest developer of voluntary international standards and it facilitates world trade by providing common standards among nations. More than twenty thousand standards have been set, covering everything from manufactured products and technology to food safety, agriculture, and healthcare.

Use of the standards aids in the creation of products and services that are safe, reliable, and of good quality. The standards help businesses increase productivity while minimizing errors and waste. By enabling products from different markets to be directly compared, they facilitate companies in entering new markets and assist in the development of global trade on a fair basis. The standards also serve to safeguard consumers and the end-users of products and services, ensuring that certified products conform to the minimum standards set internationally.

History

The organization began in the 1920s as the International Federation of the National Standardizing Associations (ISA). It was suspended in 1942 during World War II, but after the war ISA was approached by the recently formed United Nations Standards Coordinating Committee (UNSCC) with a proposal to form a new global standards body. In October 1946, ISA and UNSCC delegates from 25 countries met in London and agreed to join forces to create the new International Organization for Standardization. The new organization officially began operations in February 1947.
More information can be obtained :

www.ISO.org

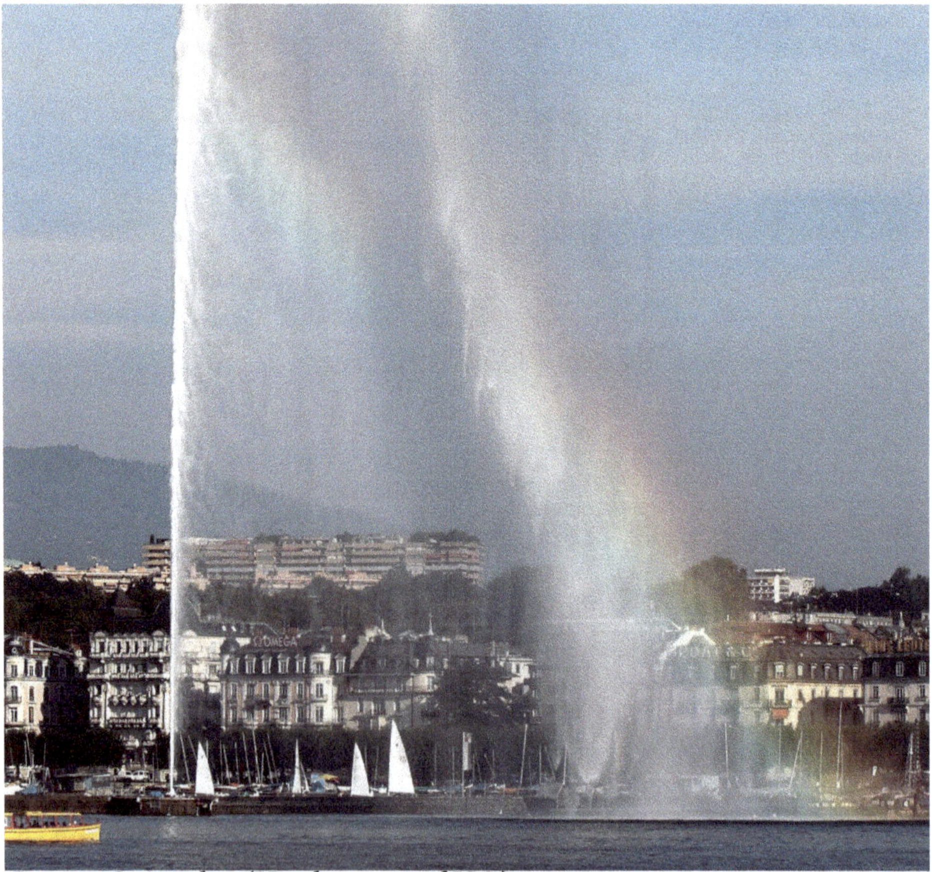

Geneva, Switzerlan (Headquarter of ISO)

CHAPTER 2

MDSAP

MDSAP The Medical Device Single Audit Program is the single audit program that covers the regulations of Australia, Brazil, Canada, Japan and USA. These regulations use the MDSAP to verify compliance to the quality systems of their national regulations and ISO 13485. The intention of the Medical Device Single Audit Program (MDSAP) is to allow competent auditors from MDSAP recognized Auditing Organizations (AOs) to conduct a single audit of a medical device organization's quality management system that will satisfy the requirements of the medical device regulatory authorities participating in the MDSAP program.

Audits performed under the MDSAP program will be process based, focusing on several defined processes, a defined method for linking those processes, and built on a foundation of requirements for risk management.

ISO 13485 MDSAP are two different programs with similar requirements but they do not duplicate each other.

MDSAP has the more stringent requirements of the two and companies that are already certified to ISO 13485 will see an increase in the number of audit days once they seek certification to MDSAP. The design of the Medical Device Single Audit Program (MDSAP) audit process is to ensure a single audit will provide efficient yet thorough coverage of regulatory requirements.

These requirements include; Medical devices – Quality management systems – Requirements for regulatory purposes (ISO 13485:2016), the Quality Management System requirements of the Conformity Assessment Procedures of the Australian Therapeutic

Goods (Medical Devices) Regulations (TG(MD)R Sch3), the Brazilian Good Manufacturing Practices (RDC ANVISA 16/2013), the Japanese Ordinance on Standards for Manufacturing Control and Quality Control of Medical Devices and In Vitro Diagnostic Reagents (MHLW Ministerial Ordinance No. 169), the Quality System Regulation (21 CFR Part 820), and specific requirements of the medical device regulatory authorities participating in the MDSAP program.

What is the meaning of ISO 13485 certified?

ISO certification is a seal of approval from a third party body that a company runs to one of the international standards developed and published by the International Organization for Standardization (ISO). ... ISO 13485 helps put your customers first.

Is ISO 13485 certification worth it?

ISO 13485 is important to designers, manufacturers, and distributors of medical devices. In addition, suppliers and service providers can enhance an organization's marketability as more and more manufacturers require certification in order to do business with a vendor.

MDSAP AUDIT:

The design and development of the MDSAP audit sequence allows a logical, focused and efficient conduct of an audit. The MDSAP audit sequence follows a process approach and has four primary processes - Management process, Measurement, Analysis and Improvement process, Design and Development process and a Production and Service Controls process with links to the supporting process for Purchasing.

The definition of each process includes a purpose and an outcome that are indicators of process performance. Each participating Regulatory Authority expects that risk management to be the foundation for the five processes that are the requirements of a quality management system for medical device organizations.

The MDSAP audit process has two additional supporting processes: Device Marketing Authorization and Facility Registration and Medical Device Adverse Events and Advisory Notices Reporting. These processes are necessary to fulfill specific requirements of the participating MDSAP regulatory authorities.

Regulatory Requirements

Country	Regulatory	MDSAP
Australia	Conformity Assessment Procedures of the Australian Therapeutic Goods (Medical Devices) Regulations (TG(MD)R Sch3)	Vo.1
Brazil	The Brazilian Good Manufacturing Practices (RDC ANVISA 2013/16)	Vol.2
Canada	Medical Devices Regulations SOR/282-98 and specific requirements of the medical device regulatory authorities	Vol.3
Japan	The Japanese Ordinance on Standards for Manufacturing Control and Quality Control of Medical Devices and In Vitro Diagnostic Reagents (MHLW Ministerial Ordinance No. 169),	Vol.4
USA	FDA Quality System Regulation (21 CFR Part 820)	Vol.5

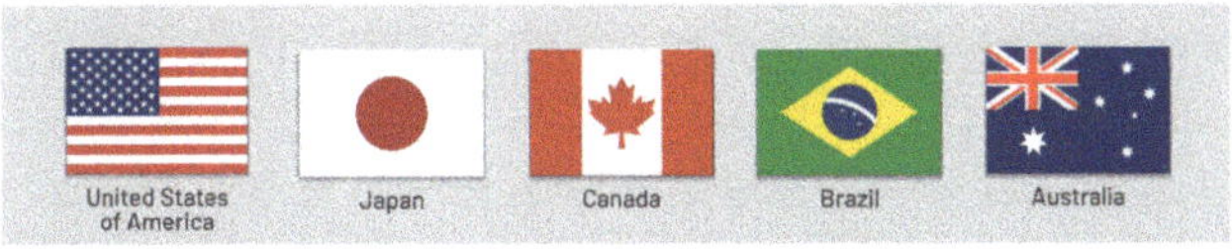

Definitions

ISO 13485 specifies requirements for a quality management system where an organization needs to demonstrate its ability to provide medical devices and related services that consistently meet customer and applicable regulatory requirements. Such organizations can be involved in one or more stages of the life-cycle, including design and development, production, storage and distribution, installation, or servicing of a medical device and design and development or provision of associated activities (e.g. technical support). ISO 13485 can also be used by suppliers or external parties that provide product, including quality management system-related services to such organizations.

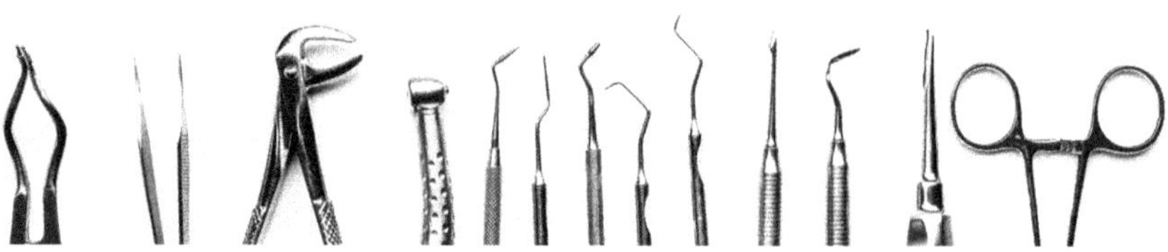

Scope of Certificate: The scope of the ISO certificate depends on how your Organization would like to have keeping in view of future. Some want to be specific by listing the products; some to be general covering the broad category of products. Here are some examples:

1. Design, development assemble, manufacture, distribute and service of life science instruments

2. Design, assemble/manufacture, sales & service of medical instruments used in cardiology including ECG Recorders, Bedside monitors

3. Design, development, manufacture, distribute and repair of medical device instruments intended to use in genetic analysis such as DNA Amplifiers, Genetic Analyzers, etc.

Distributer

Natural or legal person in the supply chain who, on his own behalf, furthers the availability of a medical device to the end user

Importer

natural or legal person in the supply chain who is the first in a supply chain to make a medical device,
manufactured in another country or jurisdiction, available in the country or jurisdiction where it is to
be marketed

Manufacturer

natural or legal person with responsibility for design and/or manufacture of a medical device with the
intention of making the medical device available for use, under his name; whether or not such a medical
device is designed and/or manufactured by that person himself or on his behalf by another person(s)

Device The term "device" is used throughout the MDSAP processes. For the purpose of applying the MDSAP processes, and to accommodate nuances in the regulatory systems of the participating Regulatory Authorities, the use of the term "device" is to refer to any product that is capable of functioning as a medical device, whether or not it is packaged, labeled, or sterilized.

Supplier: Organization or individual that enters into an agreement with the acquirer or integrator for the supply of a product or service.

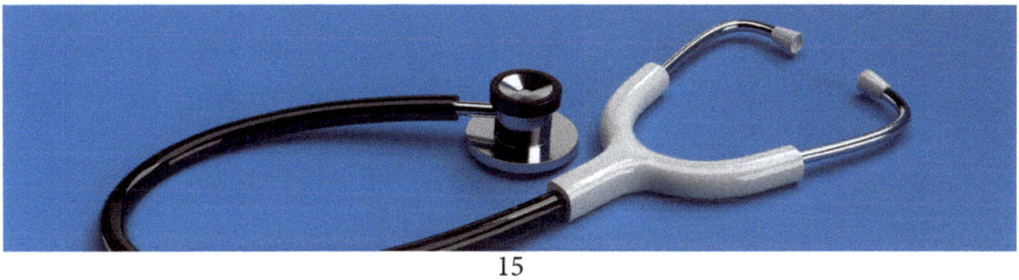

We can categorized the suppliers to:

- Critical Supplier
- Non-critical supplier

A purchased or otherwise obtained "product" or "service" is an outsourced product or service. In addition, a "supplier" is anyone that is independent from the medical device organization's quality management system. This includes a supplier that may be part of the same corporation as the medical device organization but operates under a separate quality management system from the audited medical device organization.

Critical Suppliers:

For the purposes of MDSAP, "critical suppliers" include, but are not limited to;

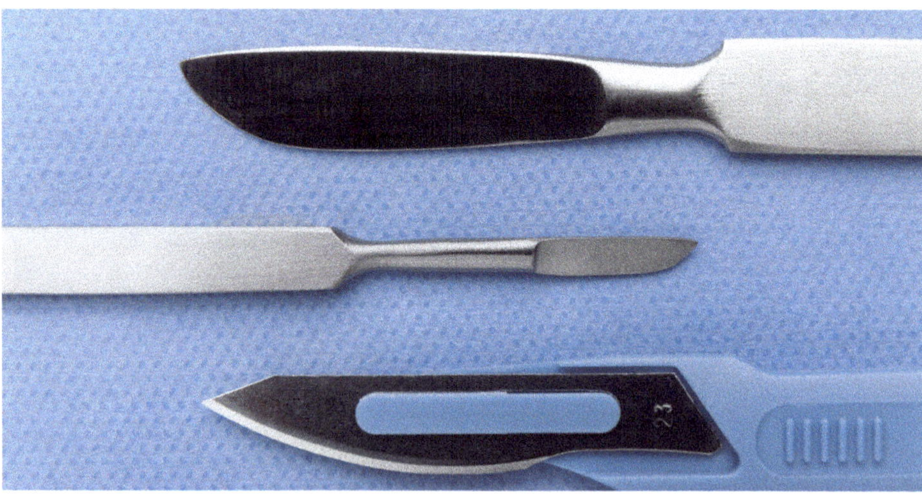

- Those entities that supply the organization with finished devices, i.e. a device, or accessory to any device, that is suitable for use or capable of functioning, whether or not it is packaged, labeled, or sterilized;
- Suppliers of products, including services, that impact design outputs that are essential for the proper functioning of the device; and
- Suppliers of products and services that require process validation.

> Not all MDSAP participating regulatory authorities require, or make use of, certification documents that relate to a medical device organization's QMS. The terms "certification" and "recertification" appear within this volumes to maintain consistency with the terminology used within ISO/IEC 17021-1:2015 Conformity assessment – Requirements for bodies providing audit and certification of management systems.

MDSAP Audit

The Medical Device Single Audit Program is based on a three (3) year audit cycle. The Initial Audit, also referred to as the "Initial Certification Audit" is a complete audit of a medical device organization's quality management system (QMS) consisting of:

Stage 1 Audit (17021-1:2015 – Cl 9.3.1.2)

Stage 2 Audit (17021-1:2015 – Cl 9.3.1.3)

The initial Audit is followed by a partial Surveillance Audit (17021-1:2015 – Cl 9.6.2.2) in each of the following two (2) years and a complete Re-audit, also referred to as a "Recertification Audit" (17021-1:2015 – Cl 9.6.3.2) in the third (3rd) year. A recertification audit may also include a Stage 1 audit if there have been significant changes to the QMS that have not been otherwise adequately assessed.

Initial Certification Audit

Initial Certification audit consists of: Stage 1 & 2

Stage 1

Documentation review, evaluation of preparedness for Stage 2 audit, etc.

A Stage 1 audit shall be conducted in accordance with Clause 9.3.1.2 of ISO/IEC 17021-1:2015 and all applicable MDSAP Audit Process tasks and regulatory requirements.

From an MDSAP perspective, the primary purposes of a Stage 1 audit are (1) to determine if QMS documentation required by ISO 13485:2016 - Clauses 4.2.1 and other applicable MDSAP documentation requirements have been adequately defined, and documented; (2) to assess the medical device organization's preparedness for a Stage 2 audit; (3) to provide a focus for planning a Stage 2 audit; and, (4) to collect information regarding the scope of the quality management system and other aspects of the medical device organization.

Portions of a Stage 1 audit (e.g. documentation review) may be performed at a site other than the site(s) of the medical device organization seeking initial certification.

The outcome of the Stage 1 audit will assist the MDSAP recognized Auditing Organization in its determination of the readiness of the medical device organization to undergo a Stage 2 audit. The Au-

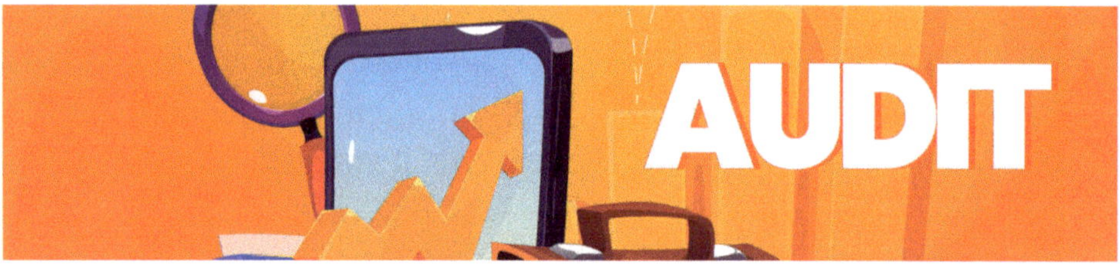

diting Organization shall determine how best to accomplish tasks of Stage 1 and Stage 2 with regards to off-site documentation and record review and on-site verifications. Hence portions of a Stage 1 audit (e.g. documentation review) may be performed at a site other than the site(s) of the medical device organization seeking initial certification. In practice it is intended that the Auditing Organization may combine elements of Stage 1 and Stage 2 to allow for a single on-site visit for the initial audit or re-audit of the medical device organization.

Stage 2

Evaluation of QMS Implementation and Effectiveness

A Stage 2 audit shall be conducted in accordance with Clause 9.3.1.3 of ISO/IEC 17021-1:2015 and using all applicable MDSAP Audit Process tasks.

The purpose of a Stage 2 audit is to determine if all applicable requirements of ISO 13485:2016 and the relevant regulatory requirements from participating regulatory authorities have been implemented. Stage 2 audit objectives shall specifically include an evaluation of:

- The effectiveness of the medical device organization's QMS incorporating the applicable regulatory requirements;
- Product/process related technologies (e.g. injection molding, sterilization);
- Adequate product technical documentation in relation to relevant regulatory requirements; and,
- The medical device organization's ability to comply with these requirements.

Surveillance Audits

(1st and 2nd Surveillance Audits):

A Surveillance Audit shall be conducted in accordance with Clause 9.6.2.2 of ISO/IEC 17021-1:2015 and clause 9.6.2 of IMDRF/MDSAP WG/N3:2016 and using applicable MDSAP Audit Process tasks. The purpose of a series of surveillance audits is to assure that all applicable requirements of ISO 13485:2016 and the relevant regulatory requirements from participating regulatory authorities are audited during the cycle of a three year audit program for the medical device organization. Surveillance audit objectives during the audit cycle shall specifically include evaluation of:

- The effectiveness of the medical device organization's QMS incorporating the applicable regulatory requirements.
- The medical device organization's ability to comply with these requirements; and
- New or changed product/process related technologies; and,
- New or amended product technical documentation in relation to relevant regulatory requirements.

In addition, surveillance audits shall include a review of issues related to medical device safety and effectiveness since the last audit such as complaints, problem reports, vigilance reports, and recalls/field corrections/advisory notices.

Re-audit (Recertification Audits)

A Re-audit (Recertification Audit) shall be conducted in accordance with Clause 9.6.3 of ISO/IEC 17021-1:2015 and using all applicable MDSAP Audit Process tasks. The purpose of a re-audit is

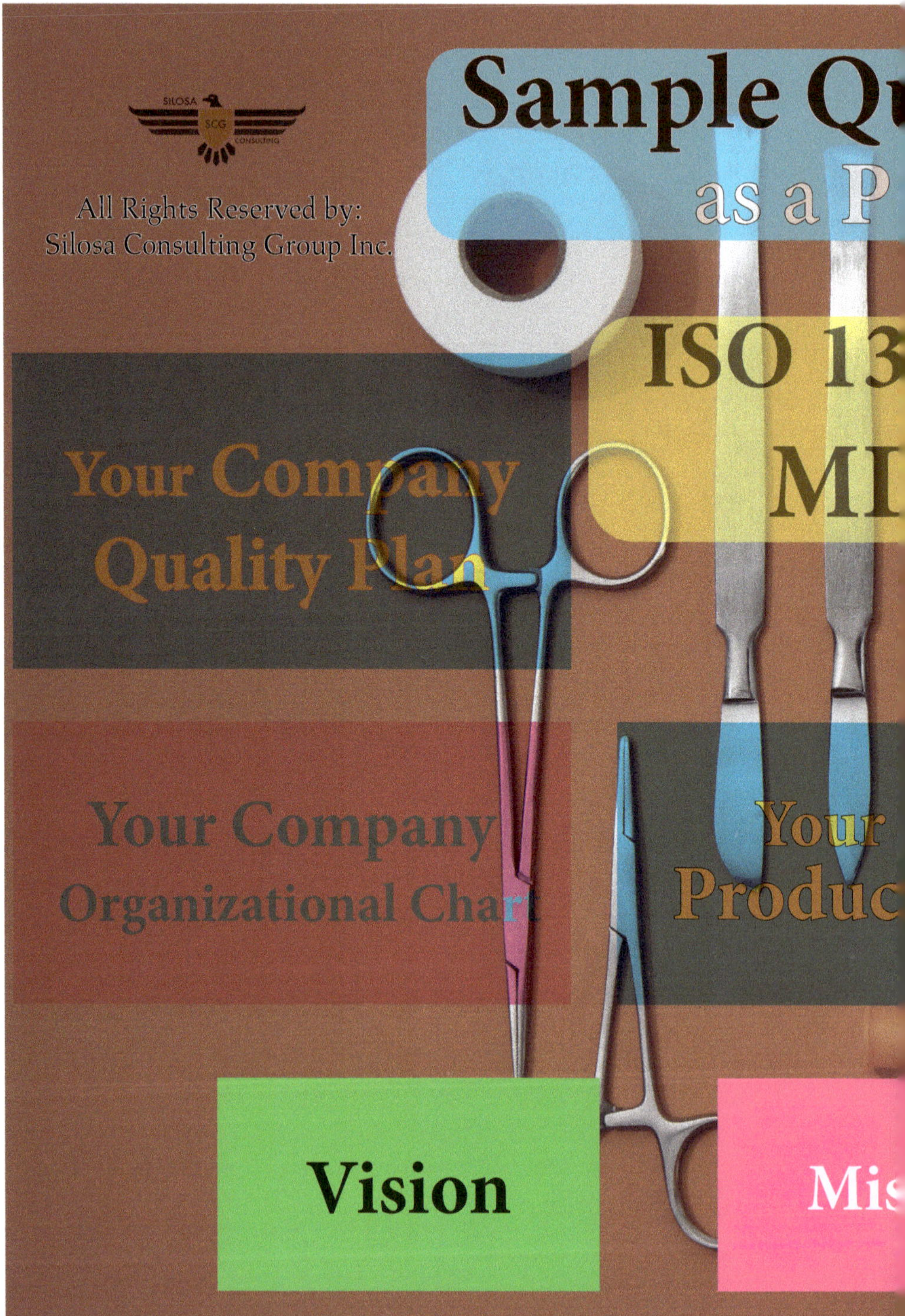
SILOSA SCG CONSULTING
All Rights Reserved by:
Silosa Consulting Group Inc.
Sample Q
as a P
ISO 13
MI
Your Company
Quality Plan
Your Company
Organizational Chart
Your
Produc
Vision
Mis

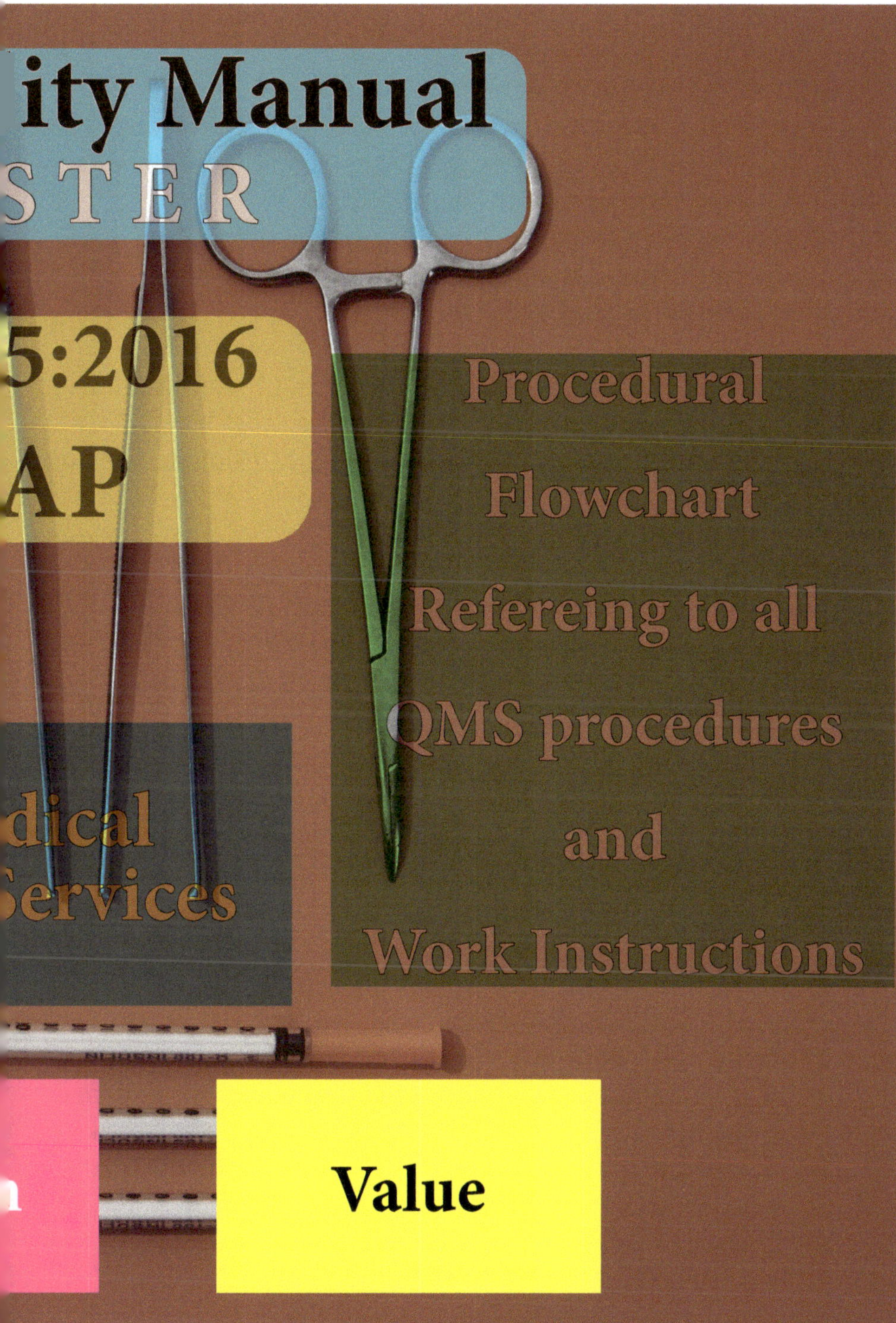
ity Manual
STER
5:2016
AP
dical
ervices
Procedural
Flowchart
Refereing to all
QMS procedures
and
Work Instructions
Value

to confirm the continued relevance, applicability and suitability of the medical device organization's QMS (as a whole), to satisfy all applicable requirements of ISO 13485:2016 and the relevant regulatory requirements from participating regulatory authorities, with respect to the scope of certification. Recertification audit objectives shall specifically include evaluation of:
- the effectiveness of the medical device organization's QMS incorporating the applicable regulatory requirements
- product/process related technologies (e.g. injection molding, sterilization)
- adequate product technical documentation in relation to relevant regulatory requirements
- the medical device organization's continued fulfillment of these requirements.

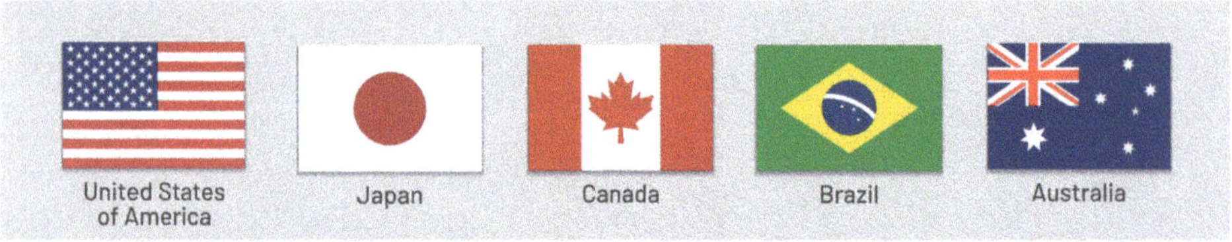

Audits Conducted by Regulatory Authorities

Audits may also be conducted by MDSAP participating regulatory authorities at any time and for a range of reasons including (1) "For Cause" due to information obtained by the regulatory authority, (2) as follow up to the findings of a previous audit, and (3) to confirm the effective implementation of MDSAP requirements by MDSAP recognized auditing organizations.

The purpose of audits conducted by regulatory authorities is to ensure appropriate oversight of a recognized MDSAP Auditing Organization's audit activities, as an alternative means of assessing medical device organizations that have been identified as undertaking high risk manufacturing processes and have not been adequately audited, where sufficient detail regarding audited processes has not been included in an audit report, or where there is a history of low compliance with QMS or regulatory requirements.

MDSAP
ISO 13485 Requirements &

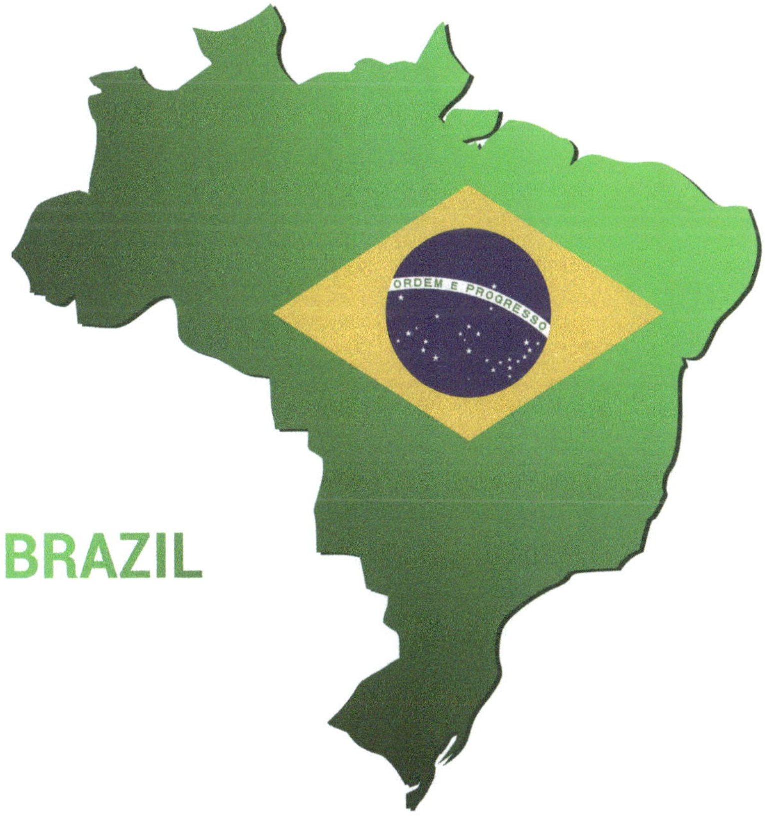

Management

The intent of the Management Process is to provide adequate resources for device design, manufacturing, quality assurance, distribution, installation, and servicing activities; to assure the quality management system is functioning properly and effectively; and to monitor the quality management system and make necessary adjustments. A quality management system that has been implemented effectively and is monitored to identify and address existing and potential problems is more likely to produce medical devices that function as intended.

The management representative is responsible for ensuring that the requirements of the quality management system have been effectively defined, documented, implemented, and maintained. Prior to the audit of a process, it may be helpful to interview the management representative (or designee) to obtain an overview of the process and a feel for management's knowledge and understanding of the process.

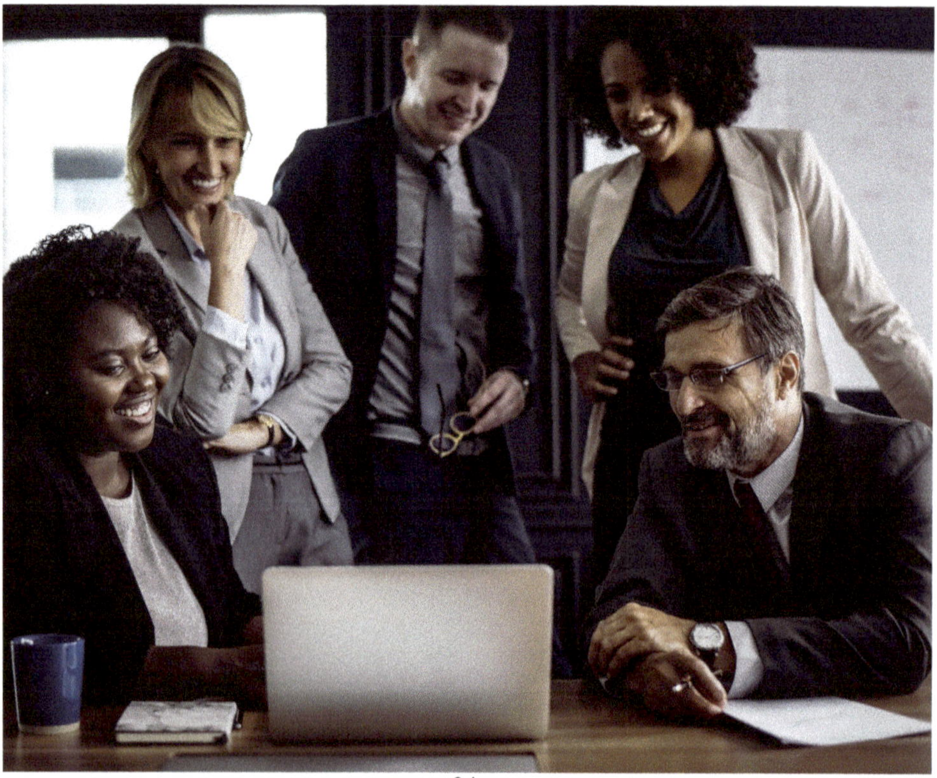

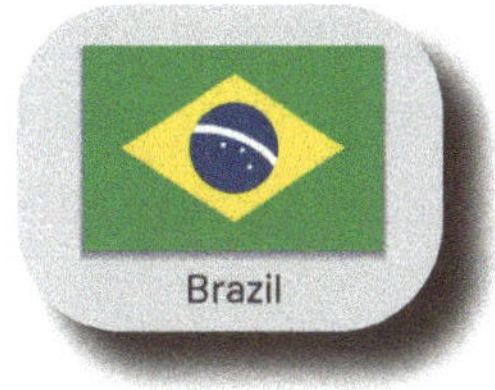

Clause and Regulation:
ISO 13485:2016: 4.1.1, 4.1.2, 4.1.3, 4.2.2, 4.1.4, 5.4.2;
ANVISA: RDC ANVISA 16/2013: 2.1, 5.6;
ANVISA: RDC ANVISA 16/2013: 2.2.5

Confirm that the manufacturer ensures that any consultant who gives advice regarding design, purchasing, manufacturing, packaging, labeling, storage, installation, or servicing of medical devices has proper qualification to perform such tasks. Those consultants shall be contracted as a formal service supplier, according to purchasing controls defined by the manufacturer [RDC ANVISA 16/2013: 2.3.3].

A review of employee training records can be performed to ensure that employees have been trained regarding the medical device organization's quality policy and objectives. In particular, this should be done for employees involved in key operations that affect product realization and product quality.

During the audit of the Production and Service Controls process, ensure that employees who are involved in key operations that affect product realization and product quality have been trained in their specific job tasks, as well as the quality policy and objectives.
When appropriate, review the training records for those employees whose activities have contributed to process nonconformities.

When appropriate, assess the role of top management when risk-based decisions are made that appear to justify levels of risk that do not meet the medical device organization's previously established risk- acceptance criteria.

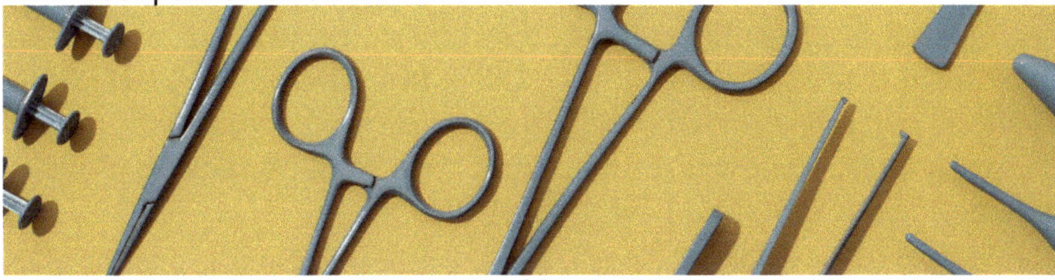

Device Marketing Authorization and Facility Registration
The Device Marketing Authorization and Facility Registration process may be audited as a linkage from the Management process and/or the Design and Development process.

Good Manufacturing Practices in Brazil

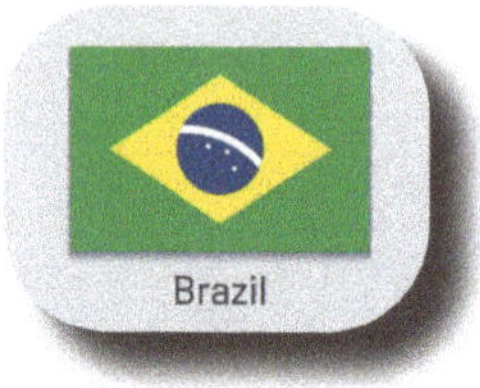

Manufacturer means any person who designs, manufactures, assembles or processes finished devices, including those who only perform sterilization process, labeling and packaging [RDC ANVISA 16/2013: 1.2.9].
For a domestic manufacturer, confirm that the establishment has ANVISA's authorization to manufacture medical devices (AFE - Autorização de Funcionamento da Empresa). For domestic and international manufacturers, verify that the products already distributed in the Brazilian market are registered/notified with ANVISA [Brazilian Federal Law nº 6360/76].
According Brazilian Legislation, the Good Manufacturing Practice (GMP) certification is a prerequisite for medical device registration. Therefore, the facility site inspection precedes the device registration request. Medical devices subject to notification do not need the GMP certificate, but even not being certified, their manufacturers shall comply with the GMP requirements.
Device marketing authorization shall be requested to ANVISA by the domestic manufacturer or importer (legal representative) formally established in Brazil. Registration is a comprehensive process for market authorization, applied to medical devices in classes III and IV. [ANVISA RDC nº 36/2015, RDC nº 40/2015]
Notification is a simplified market authorization process, applied to all medical device classes I and II. [ANVISA RDC nº 36/2015, RDC nº 40/2015]. Registration is valid for 10 years, while notification has no expiry date. Renewal of the registration shall be requested upon time defined at Brazilian Law 6360/1976.

Measurement, Analysis and Improvement

One of the most important activities in the quality management system is the identification of existing and potential causes of product and quality problems. Such causes must be identified so that appropriate and effective corrective or preventive actions can take place. These activities are carried out under the Measurement, Analysis and Improvement process.

Clause and Regulation
ISO: ISO 13485:2016: 4.2.1, 8.1, 8.2.1, 8.2.6, 8.5
ANVISA: RDC ANVISA 16/2013: 5.3.1, 7.1, 7.2

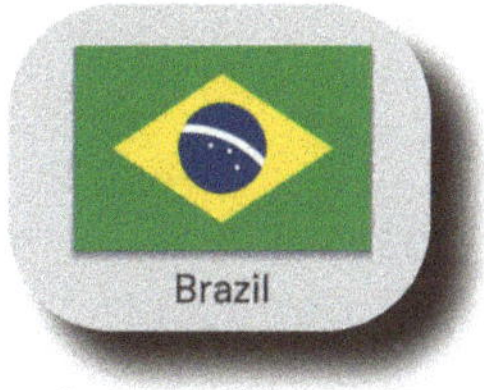

Verify that the manufacturer has ensured that information about quality problems or nonconforming products are properly disseminated to those directly involved in the maintenance of product quality and to prevent occurrence of such problems
[RDC ANVISA 16/2013: 7.1.1.6].

Verify that each manufacturer has established and maintains procedures to receive, examine, evaluate, investigate and document complaints. Such procedures must ensure that:

- Complaints are received, documented, analyzed, evaluated, investigated and documented by a formally designated unit
- Where applicable, complaints must be reported to the competent health authority
- Complaints must be examined to determine whether an investigation is necessary. When an investigation is not done, the unit must maintain a record that includes the reason that the investigation was not performed and the name of the persons responsible for the decision. Each manufacturer must examine, evaluate and investigate all complaints involving possible nonconformities of the product. Any claim for death, injury or threat to public health must be immediately reviewed, evaluated and investigated.
- The records of the investigation must include:

Product name, Date of receipt of the complaint, Any control number used, Name, address and telephone number of the complainant
Nature of complaint, Data and research results
[RDC ANVISA 16/2013: 7.2].

Medical Device Adverse Events and Advisory Notices Reporting
The Medical Device Adverse Events and Advisory Notices Reporting process may be audited as a linkage from the Measurement, Analysis and Improvement process.

Clause and Regulation
ISO: ISO 13485:2016: 4.2.1, 7.2.3, 8.2.2, 8.2.3
[RDC ANVISA 67/2009 – Art. 6°]

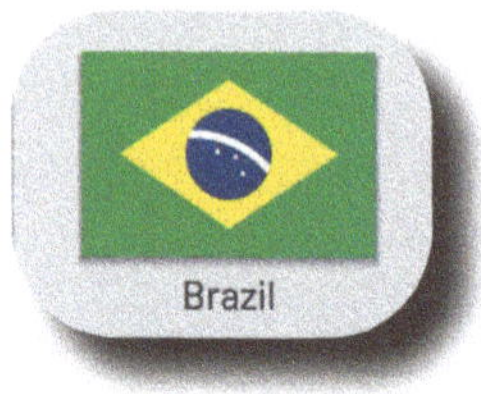

Verify that a post-market surveillance system is established and implemented in the medical device organization and integrated into the Quality System, with procedures and work flows established to ensure the correct and the prompt identification of adverse events, the performance of investigations and use of the results to improve the safety and effectiveness of the device when necessary [RDC ANVISA 67/2009 – Art. 6°].
For domestic manufacturers (also applies to legal representatives in Brazil) - verify that top management has designated a professional to be responsible for the post-market surveillance system. This designation shall be documented [RDC ANVISA 67/2009 – Art. 5°].
Verify that the medical device organization has mechanisms for processing and recording complaints, conducting investigations, and providing feedback directly to the complainant, or in the case of an international manufacturer, to their legal representative in Brazil, as necessary [RDC ANVISA 67/2009 – Art. 6°, Art. 7°, Art. 9°].
Verify that the medical device organization has notified the regulatory authority about problems associated with their devices, including adverse events (critical or non-critical), any technical defect that was identified regarding products already marketed, anything that can cause a serious hazard to public health, or cases of counterfeit [RDC ANVISA 67/2009 – Art. 8°].

For international manufacturer, verify that the legal representative in Brazil is aware about the occurrence of possibility of death, serious hazard to public health or cases of counterfeit, associated with their products exported to Brazil
[RDC ANVISA 67/2009 – Art. 8º].
Verify that procedures and work flows were established in order to identify when field actions (recalls and corrections) are necessary, in accordance with the medical device organization's post-market surveillance system and quality system [RDC ANVISA 67/2009 - Art. 6º, RDC ANVISA 23/2012 – Art. 1º, Art. 5º].
Verify that the medical device organization keeps records regarding field actions performed, including those that do not need to be reported to regulatory authorities [RDC ANVISA 23/2012 – Art. 4º; Art. 6º, Art. 10, Art. 11, Art. 16].
For domestic manufacturers (also applies to legal representatives in Brazil) - verify that the medical device organization has sent to the regulatory authority the reports requested, according Brazilian regulation [RDC ANVISA 23/2012– Art. 10, Art. 11].
Verify that the medical device organization has performed field actions based on potential or concrete evidence that their product does not comply with essential requirements of safety and effectiveness [RDC ANVISA 23/2012 – Art. 4º, Art. 6º, Art. 7º, Art. 13, Art. 14, Art. 15].
For domestic manufacturers (also applies to legal representatives in Brazil) - verify that the medical device organization has performed field actions when required by the regulatory authority [RDC ANVISA 23/2012 – Art. 6º].
For domestic manufacturers (also applies to legal representatives in Brazil) - verify that the medical device organization notified the regulatory authority regarding field actions, in accordance with requirements and deadlines established per Brazilian regulation
[RDC ANVISA 23/2012 - Art. 7º, Art. 8º].
For international manufacturers, verify that the legal representative in Brazil was aware about the occurrence of field actions performed on products exported to Brazil
[RDC ANVISA 67/2009 - Art. 8º].

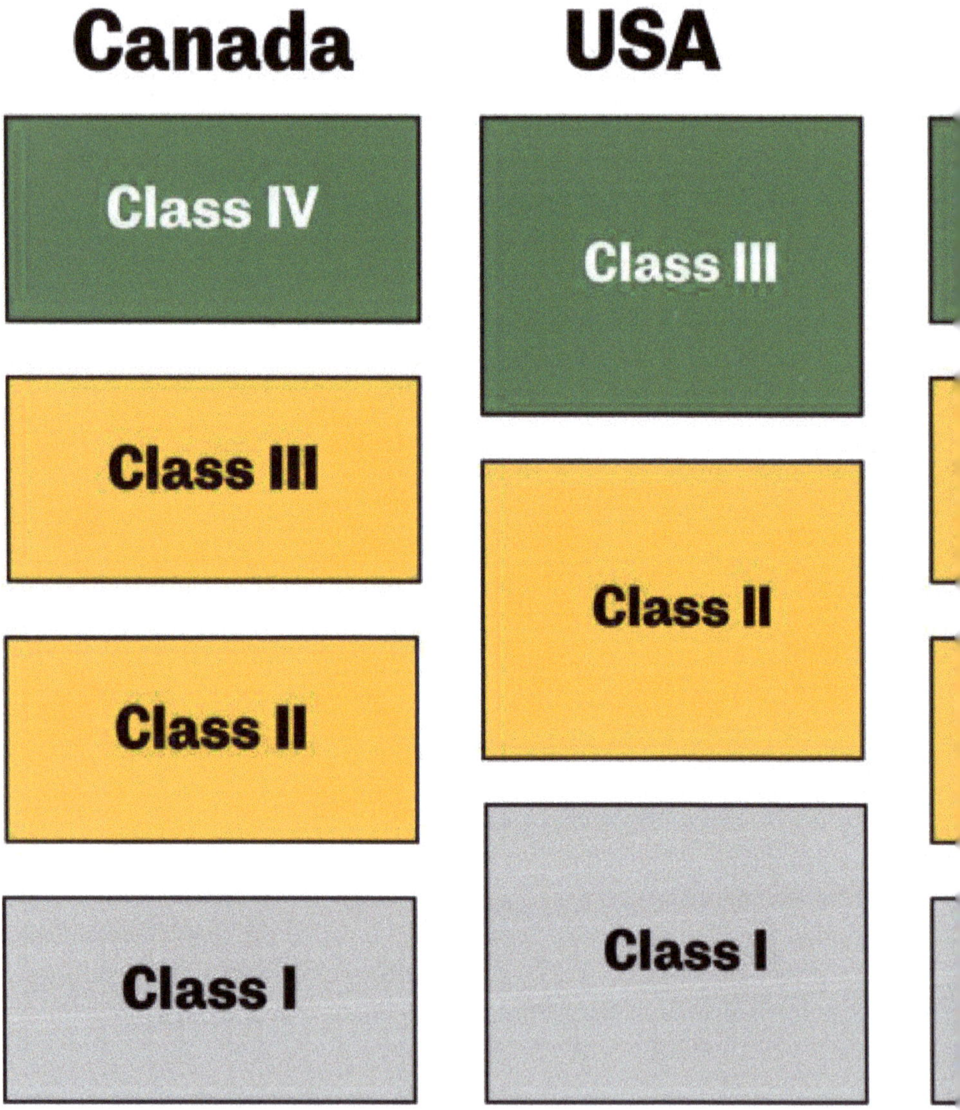
Canada
Class IV
Class III
Class II
Class I
USA
Class III
Class II
Class I

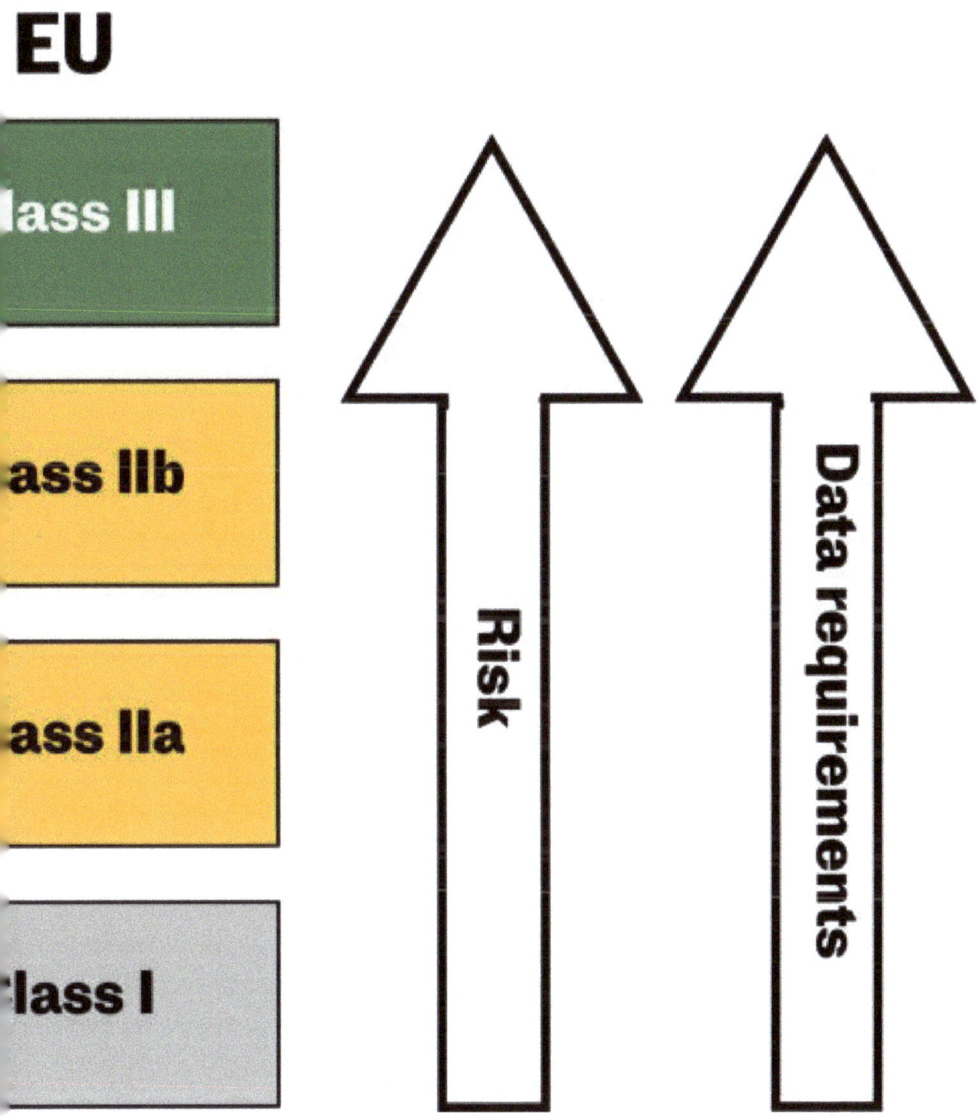
EU
lass III
ass IIb
ass IIa
lass I
Risk
Data requirements

Design and Development

The purpose of the Design and Development process is to control the design of a medical device and to assure that the device meets user needs, intended use, and its specified requirements. Attention to design and development planning, identifying design inputs, developing design outputs, verifying that design outputs meet design inputs, validating the design, controlling design changes, reviewing design results, transferring the design to production, and compiling the appropriate records will help a medical device organization assure that resulting designs will meet user needs, intended uses, and requirements. Review of the Design and Development process will also provide an opportunity to evaluate how the medical device organization has utilized risk management activities to ensure design inputs are comprehensive and meet user needs, to confirm that risk control measures that were planned have been implemented in the design, and to verify that risk control measures are effective in controlling or reducing risk.

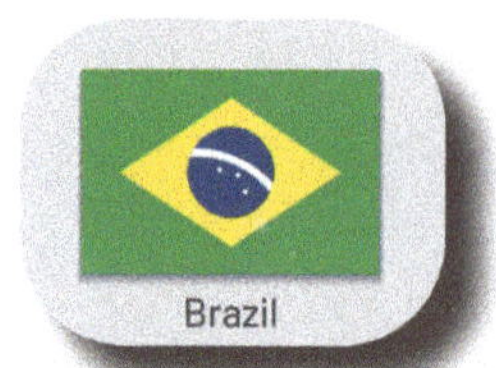

Clause and Regulation
ISO: ISO 13485:2016: 4.1.1, 4.2.1, 7.1, 7.3.10
[RDC ANVISA 16/2013: 4.1.7, 4.2].

According to Brazilian legislations, there is no exception to design control.

If design activities are outsourced, verify that the manufacturer has a complete device master record for the device and records of the design transfer to production
[RDC ANVISA 16/2013: 4.1.7, 4.2]. [RDC ANVISA 16/2013: 4.1.2, 4.1.11]

Verify that the manufacturer has established and maintains a continuous process of risk management which covers the entire life cycle of the product. Possible hazards must be identified in both normal and fault conditions, including those arising from human factors issues. The risk associated with those hazards, shall be calculated. Risks must be analyzed, evaluated and controlled, as necessary. Effectiveness of risk controls implemented shall be evaluated [RDC ANVISA 56/2001, RDC ANVISA 16/2013: 2.4].

Production and Service Controls

The purpose of the Production and Service Controls process is to manufacture products that meet specifications. Developing processes that are adequate to produce devices that meet specifications, validating (or fully verifying the results of) those processes, and monitoring and controlling those processes are all steps that help assure the result will be devices that meet specified requirements. After completing the audit of the medical device organization's Production and Service Controls process, the audit team will return to the Management process to make a final decision of whether top management ensures that an adequate and effective quality management system has been established and maintained at the medical device organization.

Clause and Regulation
ISO: ISO 13485:2016: 7.1, 7.2.1, 7.5.1
RDC ANVISA 16/2013: 2.2.1, 2.4, 4.1.2, 4.1.7, 5.1

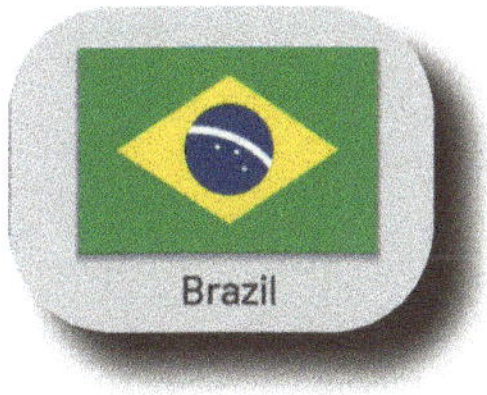

Confirm that a pest control program has been established and where chemicals are used as part of the pest control program, the company must ensure that they do not affect product quality [RDC ANVISA 16/2013: 5.1.3.4].

Verify that the manufacturer has established and maintains housekeeping procedures and schedules for production areas and warehouses, in conformance with production specifications [RDC ANVISA 16/2013: 5.1.3.1].

Verify that analytical methods, supporting auxiliary systems for production and environmental control that can adversely affect product quality or the quality system are validated, periodically reviewed and, when necessary, revalidated according to documented procedures [RDC ANVISA 16/2013: 5.5.2, 5.5.3].

Reviewing a validation

During review of a validation study, determine when applicable whether:

- The instruments used to generate the data were properly calibrated and maintained
- Predetermined product and process specifications were established
- Sampling plans used to collect test samples are based on a statistically valid rationale
- Data demonstrates predetermined specifications were met consistently
- Process tolerance limits were challenged
- Process equipment was properly installed, adjusted, and maintained
- Process monitoring instruments were properly calibrated and maintained
- Changes to the validated process were appropriately challenged (if applicable)
- Process operators were appropriately qualified.

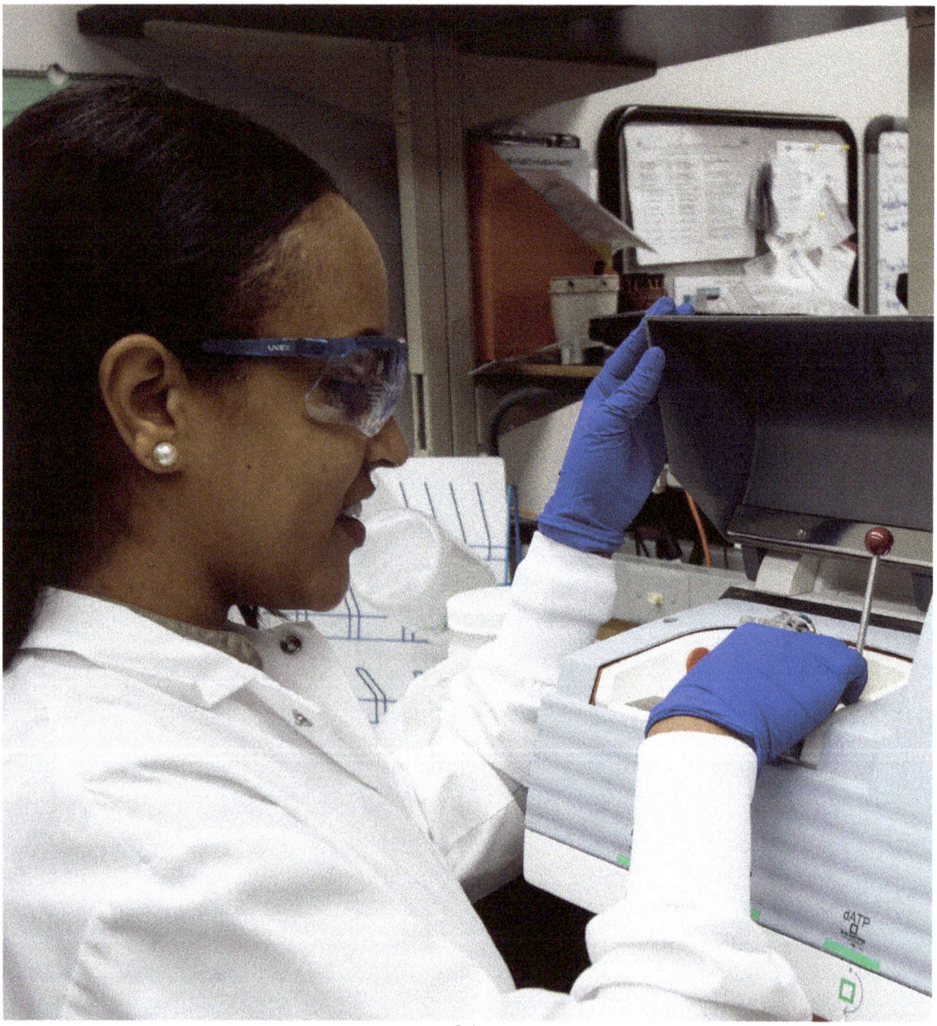

Purchasing

The intent of the Purchasing process is to ensure that purchased, subcontracted, or otherwise received products and services conform to specified requirements. The medical device organization is expected to establish and maintain documented controls for planning and performing purchasing activities. The controls necessary depend on the effect of the product on the quality, safety, and effectiveness of the finished device. Effective purchasing processes incorporate purchasing requirements and specifications, the selection of acceptable suppliers based on the capability of the suppliers to provide acceptable product, the performance of necessary acceptance activities, and maintenance of the required quality records.

The management representative is responsible for ensuring that the requirements of the quality management system have been effectively defined, documented, implemented, and maintained. Prior to the audit of a process, it may be helpful to interview the management representative to obtain an overview of the process and a feel for management's knowledge and understanding of the process.

Clause and Regulation
ISO: ISO: ISO 13485:2016: 4.1.2, 4.1.3, 4.1.5, 7.1, 7.4.1, 7.4.2, 7.4.3
ANVISA: RDC ANVISA16/2013: 2.5.1, 2.4

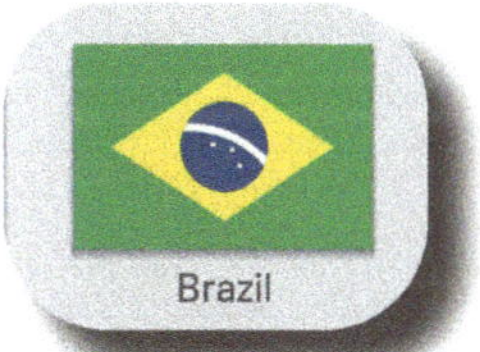

Planning

In planning product realization, the medical device organization must determine as appropriate the quality objectives and requirements for the purchased products, the processes, documents, and resources specific to the purchased products, the criteria for purchased product acceptance, and the required verification, monitoring, inspection, and test activities specific to the purchased products. Planning of product realization often begins in the design and development of the product, including the translation of the design into production specifications. The translation of the design into production specifications includes the establishment of specified requirements for purchased product.

Quality objectives

Quality objectives are typically expressed as a measurable target or goal. The planning of product realization should include consideration of how the purchased product, the criteria for purchased product acceptance, and the required verification, monitoring, inspection, and test activities specific to the purchased product will achieve the quality objectives.

- Some examples of QOB include:
- Number of complaints -v- number of parts shipped
- On-time delivery %
- Supplier parts rejected
- Comparison of internal audit findings -v- external audit findings
- Achieving a certain accuracy if you're developing product - based software
- Annual Post-market surveillance
- Auditing our system for regulatory compliance

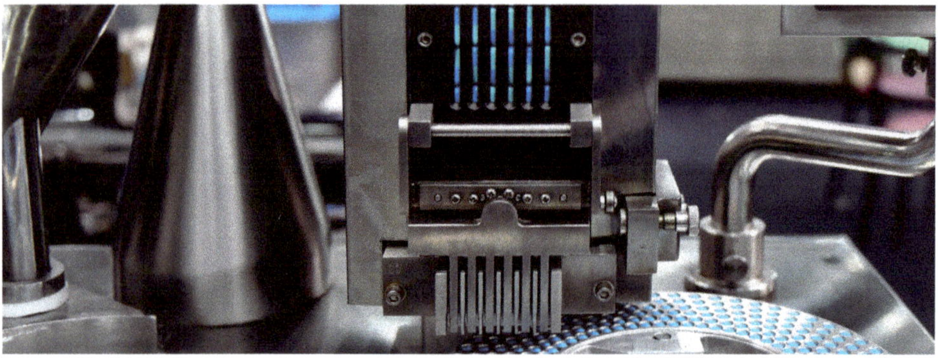

Some managers believe that the reward for hard work should be a paycheck. That's sort of like telling your children that they get to eat for doing something you're proud of. Employees are not children, but you are responsible for developing them into more valuable employees so that they can be promoted. If there is no incentive, your team will not be engaged. Therefore, pick a reward that is proportional to the bottom-line impact. Five percent of the bottom-line impact is what I like to target, but you would be amazed at how effective a few small rewards at each milestone can be. If you have trouble getting management approval for rewards, remind your boss of the bottom-line impact and link the rewards closely to the impact.

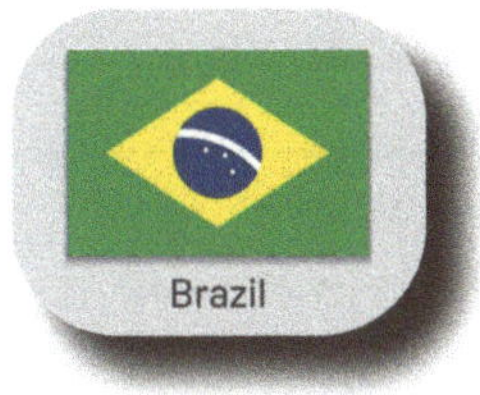

MDSAP
Audit Checklist

	REQUIREMENTS	
4 Quality management system		
4.1 General requirements		
	Has the organization:	
	a) identified the processes needed for the quality management system and their application throughout the organization (see 1.2)?	
	b) determined the sequence and interaction of these processes?	
	c) determined criteria and methods needed to ensure that both the operation and control of these processes are effective?	
	d) ensured the availability of resources and information necessary to support the operation and monitoring of their processes?	
	e) monitored, measured, and analyzed these processes	
	f) implemented actions necessary to achieve planned results and maintain the effectiveness of these processes?	
	Does the organization manage these processes in accordance with the requirements of this International Standard?	
	Where an organization chooses to outsource any process that affects product conformity with requirements, does the organization ensure control over such processes?	
	Is the control of such outsourced processes identified within the quality management system? (see 8.5.1)	
4.2.1 General		

Doc. Reference	Adequate?	Stage I (clauses marked *)	Stage II
	Y/N	Initial›s	Initial›s

	REQUIREMENTS	
	Does the quality management system documentation include:	
	a) documented statements of a quality policy and quality objectives?	
	b) a quality manual?	
	c) documented procedures required by this international standard?	
	d) documents needed by the organization to ensure the effective planning, operation and control of its processes?	
	e) records required by this International Standard (see 4.2.4)?	
	f) any other documentation specified by national or regional regulations?	
	Has the organization established and maintained a file for each type or model of medical device either containing or identifying documents defining product specifications and quality system requirements (see 4.2.3)?	
	Do these documents define the complete manufacturing process and, if applicable, installation and servicing?	
Brazil	According to Brazilian legislations, there is no exception to design control. If design activities are outsourced, verify that the manufacturer has a complete device master record for the device and records of the design transfer to production [RDC ANVISA 4.2 ,4.1.7 :2013/16].	
Brazil	Verify that the manufacturer maintains distribution records which include or make reference to: the name and address of the consignee, the identification and quantity of products shipped, the date of dispatch, and any numerical control used for traceability [RDC ANVISA 6.3 :2013/16].	

Doc. Reference	Adequate?	Stage I (clauses marked *)	Stage II
		*	

	REQUIREMENTS
EU	Does the file contain or refer to the location of objective evidence establishing the safety and effectiveness of the device as required by Annex 1 of the MDD? (MDD Annex I)
4.2.2 Quality manual	
	Has the organization established and maintained a quality manual that includes:
	a) the scope of the quality management system, including details of and justification for any exclusion and/or non-application (see 1.2)?
	b) the documented procedures established for the quality management system, or reference to them?
	c) a description of the interaction between the processes of the quality management system?
	Does the quality manual outline the structure of the documentation used in the quality management system?
Brazil	For domestic manufacturers, confirm that the establishment has ANVISA's authorization to manufacture medical devices (AFE - Autorização de Funcionamento da Empresa.)
	For domestic and international manufacturers, verify that the products already distributed in the Brazilian market, are registered/notified with ANVISA [Brazilian Federal Law 76/6360].
EU	Are the applicable sections of the Medical Device Directive (MDD) included in the specified requirements throughout the documented quality system? Interpretation: A statement only indicating compliance/conformity with the relevant international or EU regulatory requirements is not acceptable.
4.2.3 Control of documents	
	Are documents required by the quality management system controlled?

	Doc. Reference	Adequate?	Stage I (clauses marked *)	Stage II

	REQUIREMENTS	
	Is a documented procedure established to define the controls needed:	
	a) To review and approve documents for adequacy prior to issue?	
	b) To review and update as necessary and re-approve documents?	
	c) To ensure that changes and the current revision status of documents are identified?	
	d) To ensure that relevant versions of applicable documents are available at points of use?	
	e) To ensure the documents remain legible and readily identifiable?	
	f) To ensure that documents of external origin are identified and their distribution controlled?	
	g) To prevent the unintended use of obsolete documents and to apply suitable identification to them if they are retained for any purpose?	
	Does the organization ensure that changes to documents are reviewed and approved either by the original approving function or another designated function which has access to pertinent background information upon which to base its decisions?	
	Does the organization define the period for which at least one copy of obsolete controlled documents shall be retained?	
	Does this period ensure that documents to which medical devices have been manufactured and tested are available for at least the lifetime of the medical device as defined by the organization, but not less than the retention period of any resulting record (see 4.2.4), or as specified by relevant regulatory requirements?	

Doc. Reference	Adequate?	Stage I (clauses marked *)	Stage II

	REQUIREMENTS
Brazil	Verify that change records include a description of the change, identification of the affected documents, the signature of the approving individual(s), the approval date, and when the change becomes effective [RDC ANVISA 3.1.5 :2013/16]. Confirm that the manufacturer maintains a master list of the approved and effective documents [RDC ANVISA :2013/16 3.1.5]. Verify that electronic records and documents have backups [RDC ANVISA 3.1.6 :2013/16].
4.2.4 Control of quality records	
	Are records established and maintained to provide evidence of conformity to requirements and of the effective operation of the quality management system?
	Do records remain legible, readily identifiable and retrievable?
	Has a documented procedure been established to define the controls needed for the identification, storage, protection, retrieval, retention time and disposition of records?
	Does the organization retain the records for a period of time at least equivalent to the lifetime of the medical device as defined by the organization, but not less than two years from the date of product release by the organization or as specified by relevant regulatory requirements?
EU	Has the manufacturer retained for a period ending at least five years after the last product has been manufactured, the records listed in Annex II, 6.1 or Annex V, 5.1 or Annex VI, 5.1 (whichever applies)
5 Management responsibility	
5.1 Management commitment	

Doc. Reference	Adequate?	Stage I (clauses marked *)	Stage II

	REQUIREMENTS	
	Has top management provided evidence of its commitment to the development and implementation of the quality management system and maintaining its effectiveness by:	
	a) Communicating to the organization the importance of meeting customer as well as statutory and regulatory requirements?	
	b) Establishing the quality policy?	
	c) Ensuring that quality objectives are established?	
	d) Conducting management reviews?	
	e) Ensuring the availability of resources?	
5.2 Customer focus		
	Does top management ensure that customer requirements are determined and met (see 7.2.1 and 8.2.1)?	
5.3 Quality policy		
	Does top management ensure that the quality policy	
	a) Is appropriate to the purpose of the organization?	
	b) Includes a commitment to comply with requirements and to maintain the effectiveness of the quality management system?	
	c) Provides a framework for establishing and reviewing quality objectives?	
	d) Is communicated and understood within the organization?	
	e) Is reviewed for continuing suitability?	
5.4 Planning		
5.4.1 Quality objectives		
	Does top management ensure that quality objectives, including those needed to meet requirements for product (see 7.1a), are established at relevant functions and levels within the organization?	
	Are quality objectives measurable?	

Doc. Reference	Adequate?	Stage I (clauses marked *)	Stage II

	REQUIREMENTS	
	Are quality objectives consistent with the quality policy?	
5.4.2 Quality management system planning		
	Has top management ensured that:	
	a) The planning of the quality management system is carried out in order to meet the requirements given in 4.1, as well as the quality objectives?	
	b) The integrity of the quality management system is maintained when changes to the quality management system are planned and implemented?	
5.5 Responsibility, authority and communication		
5.5.1 Responsibility and authority		
	Has top management ensured that responsibilities and authorities were defined, documented and communicated within the organization?	
	Has top management established the interrelation of all personnel who manage, perform and verify work affecting quality, and ensured the independence and authority necessary to perform these tasks?	
5.5.2 Management representative		
	Has top management appointed a member of management who, irrespective of other responsibilities, has responsibility and authority that includes:	
	a) Ensuring that processes needed for the quality management system are established, implemented, and maintained?	
	b) Reporting to top management on the performance of the quality management system and any need for improvement (see 8.5)?	
	c) Ensuring the promotion of awareness of regulatory and customer requirements throughout the organization?	
5.5.3 Internal communication		

Doc. Reference	Adequate?	Stage I (clauses marked *)	Stage II

	REQUIREMENTS	
	Has top management ensured that appropriate communication processes have been established within the organization and that communication takes place regarding the effectiveness of the quality management system?	
5.6 Management review		
5.6.1 General		
	Does top management review the organization's quality management system, at planned intervals, to ensure its continuing suitability, adequacy and effectiveness?	
	Does this review include assessing opportunities for improvement and the need for changes to the quality management system, including the quality policy and quality objectives?	
	Are records from management reviews maintained (see 4.2.4)?	
5.6.2 Review input		
	Does the input to management review include information on:	
	a) Results of audits?	
	b) Customer feedback?	
	c) Process performance and product conformity?	
	d) Status of preventive and corrective actions?	
	e) Follow-up actions from previous management reviews?	
	f) Changes that could affect the quality management system?	
	g) Recommendations for improvement?	
	h) New or revised regulatory requirements?	
Brazil	Confirm that relevant information about quality problems is identified and corrective and preventive actions are submitted to executive management for information and monitoring, as well as the competent health authority, if applicable [RDC ANVISA 7.1.1.7 :2013/16].	

Doc. Reference	Adequate?	Stage I (clauses marked *)	Stage II

	REQUIREMENTS	
5.6.3 Review output		
	Does output from the management review include any decisions and actions related to:	
	a) Improvements needed to maintain the effectiveness of the quality management system and its processes?	
	b) Improvement of product related to customer requirements?	
	c) Resource needs?	
6 Resource management		
6.1 Provision of resources		
	Does the organization determine and provide the resources needed:	
	a) To implement the quality management system and to maintain its effectiveness?	
	b) To meet regulatory and customer requirements?	
6.2 Human resources		
6.2.1 General		
	Are personnel performing work affecting product quality competent on the basis of appropriate education, training, skills and experience?	
6.2.2 Competence, awareness and training		

Doc. Reference	Adequate?	Stage I (clauses marked *)	Stage II

	REQUIREMENTS	
	Does the organization:	
	a) determine the necessary competence for personnel performing work affecting product quality?	
	b) Provide training or take other actions to satisfy these needs?	
	c) Evaluate the effectiveness of actions taken?	
	d) Ensure that its personnel are aware of the relevance and importance of their activities and how they contribute to the achievement of the quality objectives?	
	e) Maintain appropriate records of education, training, skills and experience (see 4.2.4)?	
Brazil	Confirm that the manufacturer ensures that any consultant who gives advice regarding design, purchasing, manufacturing, packaging, labeling, storage, installation, or servicing of medical devices has proper qualification to perform such tasks. Those consultants shall be contracted as a formal service supplier, according to purchasing controls defined by the manufacturer [RDC ANVISA 2.3.3 :2013/16].	
6.3 Infrastructure		
	Does the organization determine, provide and maintain the infrastructure needed to achieve conformity to product requirements?	
	Infrastructure includes, as applicable:	
	a) Buildings, workspace and associated utilities	
	b) Process equipment, both hardware and software	
	c) Supporting services such as transport or communication	
	Does the organization establish documented requirements for maintenance activities, including their frequency, when such activities or lack thereof can affect product quality?	
	Are records of such maintenance maintained (see 4.2.4)?	

Doc. Reference	Adequate?	Stage I (clauses marked *)	Stage II

	REQUIREMENTS	
Brazil	Verify that manufacturing facilities are configured in order to provide adequate means for production, avoid mix-ups or contamination of components, raw materials, in process products and finished devices; and to ensure the correct handling of the devices and production flow [RDC ANVISA 5.1.2 :2013/16].	
	Has the organization determined and does it manage the work environment needed to achieve conformity to product requirements?	
	a) Has the organization established documented requirements for health, cleanliness and clothing of personnel if contact between such personnel and the product or work environment could adversely affect the quality of the product (see 7.5.1.2.1)?	
	b) If work environment conditions can have an adverse effect on product quality, has organization established documented requirements for the work environment conditions and documented procedures or work instructions to monitor and control these work environment conditions (see 7.5.1.2.1)?	
	c) Does the organization ensure that all personnel who are required to work temporarily under special environmental conditions within the work environment are appropriately trained or supervised by a trained person [see 6.2.2 b)]?	
	d) If appropriate, are special arrangements established and documented for the control of contaminated or potentially contaminated product in order to prevent contamination of other product, the work environment or personnel (see 7.5.3.1)?	
Brazil	Verify that biosafety standards are used, when applicable [RDC ANVISA 5.1.3.6 :2013/16].	

Doc. Reference	Adequate?	Stage I (clauses marked *)	Stage II
NA			

	REQUIREMENTS	
7 Product realization		
7.1 Planning of product realization		
	Has the organization planned and developed the processes needed for product realization?	
	Is the planning of product realization consistent with the requirements of the other processes of the quality management system (see 4.1)?	
	In planning product realization, has the organization determined the following, as appropriate:	
	a) Quality objectives and requirements for products?	
	b) The need to establish processes, documents, and provide resources specific to the product?	
	c) Required verification, validation, monitoring, inspection and test activities specific to the product and the criteria for product acceptance?	
	d) Records needed to provide evidence that the realization processes and resulting product meet requirements (see 4.2.4)?	
	Is the output of this planning in a form suitable for the organization's method of operations?	
	Does the organization establish documented requirements for risk management throughout product realization and are records arising from risk management maintained (see 4.2.4)?	

Doc. Reference	Adequate?	Stage I (clauses marked *)	Stage II

	REQUIREMENTS
Brazil	Verify that the manufacturer has established and maintains a continuous process of risk management which covers the entire life cycle of the product. Possible hazards must be identified in both, normal and fault conditions, including those arising from human factors issues. The risk associated with those hazards, shall be calculated. Risks must be analyzed, evaluated and controlled, as necessary. Effectiveness of risk controls implemented shall be evaluated [RDC ANVISA 2001/56 :2013/16, RDC ANVISA :2013/16 2.4].
EU	Does the supplier evaluate the need for risk analysis throughout the design process and maintain records of any risk analysis performed? (MDD Annex 1)

Doc. Reference	Adequate?	Stage I (clauses marked *)	Stage II

	REQUIREMENTS
Brazil	Verify that procedures ensure that the device design is correctly translated into production specifications [RDC ANVISA 4.1.7 :2013/16]. Confirm that the manufacturer ensures that the design release occurs only after the approval(s) of a designated person. Before the final release, design and development records must be reviewed to confirm that the design is complete and that the final design meets the approved design. Final release, including signature(s) (manual or electronic) and dates, shall be documented [RDC ANVISA 4.1.11 ,4.1.9 :2013/16]. Verify that production specifications are documented (e.g. Device Master Record – DMR). The record shall include or make reference to: a) device specifications, including software source code (if applicable), drawings, composition (BOM – bill of materials), etc.; b) production specifications (ex. work instructions, environmental controls, measurement equipment, etc.); c) labeling and packaging specifications; c) measurements, inspections, and tests, with acceptance criteria; and d) methods and procedures for installation and servicing (if applicable) [RDC ANVISA 4.2 :2013/16].
7.2.1 Determination of requirements related to the product	
	Has the organization determined:
	a) Requirements specified by the customer, including the requirements for delivery and post-delivery activities?
	b) Requirements not stated by the customer but necessary for specified or intended use, where known?
	c) Statutory and regulatory requirements related to the product?
	d) Any additional requirements determined by the organization?

Doc. Reference	Adequate?	Stage I (clauses marked *)	Stage II

	REQUIREMENTS
Brazil	Verifiy for domestic and international manufacturers that the products already distributed in the Brazilian market are registered/notified with ANVISA [Brazilian Federal Law nº 76/6360]. • Medical devices registration/notification: Device marketing authorization shall be requested to ANVISA by the domestic manufacturer or importer (legal representative) formally established in Brazil. Registration is a comprehensive process for market authorization, applied to medical devices in classes III and IV, and some class I and II devices, listed on an exception list [ANVISA IN nº 2011/03]. Notification is a simplified market authorization process, applied to medical device classes I and II, not listed on the exception list [ANVISA IN nº 2011/03]. Both registration and notification are valid for 5 years – renewal of these authorizations shall be requested upon time defined at Brazilian Law 1976/6360. • Establishment license: Domestic manufacturer: shall be authorized by ANVISA, at a minimum, as a manufacturer of medical devices. This license includes authorization to store and distribute medical devices. Importer: the importer is considered the legal representative of the international manufacturer in Brazil and shall be authorized by ANVISA to import, store, and distribute medical devices.

Doc. Reference	Adequate?	Stage I (clauses marked *)	Stage II

	REQUIREMENTS	
EU	Vefiy that manufacturing maintains files containing or refer to the location of objective evidence establishing the safety and effectiveness of the device as required by Annex 1 of the MDD. Verify that the manufacturer followed a defined and effective process to establish and maintain a file containing documents defining product specifications and quality system requirements for each newa and existing type/modes of medical devices. Since the last audit, has the manufacturer introduced new products in the EU? Has the manufacturer followed a defined and effective process to obtain an approval from the Notified Body to CE mark a product prior to selling it in the EU? (does not apply to class I devices)	
7.2.2 Review of requirements related to the product		
	Does the organization review the requirements related to the product?	
	Is this review conducted prior to the organization's commitment to supply a product to the customer (e.g. submission of tenders, acceptance of contracts or orders, acceptance of changes to contracts or orders)?	
	Does the organization ensure that:	
	a) Product requirements are defined and documented?	
	b) Contract or order requirements differing from those previously expressed are resolved?	
	c) The organization has the ability to meet the defined requirements?	
	Are records of the results of the review and actions arising from the review maintained (see 4.2.4)?	

Doc. Reference	Adequate?	Stage I (clauses marked *)	Stage II

	REQUIREMENTS	
	Where the customer provides no documented statement of requirement, are the customer requirements confirmed by the organization before acceptance?	
	Where product requirements are changed, does the organization ensure that relevant documents are amended and that relevant personnel are made aware of the changed requirements?	
7.2.3 Customer communication		
	Has the organization determined and implemented effective arrangements for communicating with customers in relation to:	
	a) Product information?	
	b) Enquiries, contracts or order handling, including amendments?	
	c) Customer feedback, including customer complaints? (see 8.2.1)	
	d) Advisory notices? (see 8.5.1)	
7.3 Design and development		
7.3.1 Design and/or development planning		
	Has the organization established documented procedures for design and development?	
	Does the organization plan and control the design and development of product?	
	During the design and development planning, does the organization determine:	
	a) The design and development stages?	
	b) The review, verification, validation and design transfer activities (see Note) that are appropriate at each design and development stage?	
	c) The responsibilities and authorities for design and development?	

Doc. Reference	Adequate?	Stage I (clauses marked *)	Stage II

	REQUIREMENTS	
	Does the organization manage the interfaces between different groups involved in design and development to ensure effective communication and clear assignment of responsibility?	
	Is planning output documented, and updated as appropriate, as the design and development progresses? (See 4.2.3)	
7.3.2 Design and development inputs		
	Have inputs relating to product requirements been determined and records maintained (see 4.2.4)?	
	Do these inputs include:	
	a) Functional, performance and safety requirements, according to the intended use?	
	b) Applicable statutory and regulatory requirements?	
	c) Where applicable, information derived from previous similar designs?	
	d) Other requirements essential for design and development?	
	e) Output(s) of risk management (see 7.1)?	
	Are these inputs reviewed for adequacy and approved?	
	Are requirements complete, unambiguous and not in conflict with each other?	
7.3.3 Design and development outputs		
	Are the outputs of design and development provided in a form that enables verification against the design and development input, and is it approved prior to release?	

Doc. Reference	Adequate?	Stage I (clauses marked *)	Stage II

	REQUIREMENTS	
	Do design and development outputs:	
	a) meet the input requirements for design and development?	
	b) Provide appropriate information for purchasing, production and for service provision?	
	c) Contain or reference product acceptance criteria?	
	d) Specify the characteristics of the product that are essential for its safe and proper use?	
	Are records of the design and development outputs maintained (see 4.2.4)?	
7.3.4 Design and development review		
	At suitable stages, are systematic reviews of design and development performed in accordance with planned arrangements (see 7.3.1):	
	a) To evaluate the ability of the results of design and development to meet requirements?	
	b) To identify any problems and propose necessary actions?	
	Do participants in such reviews include representatives of functions concerned with the design and development stage(s) being reviewed, as well as other specialist personnel (see 5.5.1 and 6.2.1)?	
	Are records of the results of the reviews and any necessary actions maintained (see 4.2.4)?	
EU	Does the supplier evaluate the need for risk analysis throughout the design process and maintain records of any risk analysis performed? (MDD Annex 1)	
7.3.5 Design and development verification		
	Is verification performed in accordance with planned arrangements (see 7.3.1) to ensure that the design and development outputs have met the design and development input requirements?	
	Are records of the results of the verification and any necessary actions maintained?	

Doc. Reference	Adequate?	Stage I (clauses marked *)	Stage II

	REQUIREMENTS	
7.3.6 Design and development validation		
	Is design and development validation performed in accordance with planned arrangements (see 7.3.1) to ensure that the resulting product is capable of meeting the requirements for the specified application or intended use?	
	Is validation completed prior to the delivery or implementation of the product (see Note 1)?	
	Are records of the results of validation and any necessary actions maintained (see 4.2.4)?	
	As part of design and development validation, does the organization perform clinical evaluations and/or evaluation of performance of the medical device, as required by national or regional regulations (see Note 2)?	
Brazil	Verify that design validation has been performed under defined operating conditions on initial production units, lots, or batches. Validation shall include device testing under real or simulated conditions of use. Design validation shall include software validation, as necessary. Stability studies shall be performed as necessary [RDC ANVISA :2013/16 4.1.8].	
7.3.7 Control of design and development changes		
	Are design and development changes identified and records maintained?	
	Are changes reviewed, verified, and validated, as appropriate, and approved before implementation?	
	Does the review of design and development changes include evaluation of the effect of the changes on constituent parts and product already delivered?	
	Are records of the results of the review of changes and any necessary actions maintained?	

Doc. Reference	Adequate?	Stage I (clauses marked *)	Stage II

	REQUIREMENTS
Brazil	If the medical device evaluated is already registered/notified with ANVISA, verify that the design change was correctly and promptly submitted to ANVISA for approval, when applicable [Brazilian Law 76/6360 - Art. 13].
EU	Do documented procedures identify the need to report essential changes to the Notified Body, (MDD Annex II, V, VI, 3.4)
7.4 Purchasing	
7.4.1 Purchasing process	
	Has the organization established documented procedures to ensure that purchased product conforms to specified purchase requirements?
	Is the type and extent of control applied to the supplier and the purchased product dependent upon the effect of the purchased product on subsequent product realization or the final product?
	Does the organization evaluate and select suppliers based on their ability to supply product in accordance with the organization's requirements?
	Have criteria for selection, evaluation and re-evaluation been established?
	Are records of the results of evaluation and any necessary actions arising from the evaluation maintained (see 4.2.4)?
Brazil	Confirm that the manufacturer establishes and maintains records of approved suppliers, contractors, and consultants [RDC ANVISA 2.5.3 ,2.3.3 :2013/16].

Doc. Reference	Adequate?	Stage I (clauses marked *)	Stage II

	REQUIREMENTS	
7.4.2 Purchasing information		
	Does purchasing information describe the product to be purchased, including where appropriate:	
	a) Requirements for approval of product, procedures, processes and equipment?	
	b) Requirements for qualification of personnel?	
	c) Quality management system requirements?	
	Does the organization ensure the adequacy of specified purchase requirements prior to their communication to the supplier?	
	To the extent required for traceability given in 7.5.3.2, does the organization maintain relevant purchasing information, i.e. documents (see 4.2.3) and records (see 4.2.4)?	
Brazil	Confirm that an agreement is established and documented in which suppliers agree to notify the manufacturer of any change in the product or service, so that the manufacturer can determine whether the change affects the quality of the finished product [RDC ANVISA 2.5.5 :2013/16].	
7.4.3 Verification of purchased product		
	Has the organization established and implemented the inspection or other activities necessary for ensuring that purchased product meets specified purchase requirements?	
	Where the organization or its customer intends to perform verification at the supplier's premises, does the organization state the intended verification arrangements and method of product release in the purchasing information?	
	Are records of the verification maintained (see 4.2.4)?	
Brazil	Verify that the manufacturer has established and maintains procedures to ensure the retention of components, raw materials, in-process products and returned products until inspections, tests or other specified verifications have been performed and documented [RDC ANVISA 5.3.3 :2013/16].	

Doc. Reference	Adequate?	Stage I (clauses marked *)	Stage II

	REQUIREMENTS	
7.5 Production and service provision		
7.5.1 Control of production and service provision		
7.5.1.1 General Requirements		
	Does the organization plan and carry out production and service provision under controlled conditions?	
	Do the controlled conditions include, as applicable:	
	a) The availability of information that describes the characteristics of the product?	
	b) The availability of documented procedures, documented requirements, work instructions, reference materials and reference measurement procedures as necessary?	
	c) The use of suitable equipment?	
	d) The availability and use of monitoring and measuring devices?	
	e) The implementation of monitoring and measurement?	
	f) The implementation of release, delivery and post-delivery activities?	
	g) The implementation of defined operations for labeling and packaging?	
	Does the organization establish and maintain a record (see 4.2.4) for each batch of medical devices that provides traceability to the extent specified in 7.5.3 and identifies the amount manufactured and amount approved for distribution?	
	Is the batch record verified and approved?	

Doc. Reference	Adequate?	Stage I (clauses marked *)	Stage II

	REQUIREMENTS
Brazil	Determine whether the manufacturer has established and maintained a procedure for change control in order to track changes in auxiliary systems, software, equipment, processes, methods or other changes that may affect the quality of products, including risk assessment within the risk management process. The procedure must describe the actions to be taken, including, when appropriate, the need for re-qualification or re-validation. Verify that changes are formally requested, documented and approved before implementation [RDC ANVISA 5.6.2 ;5.6.1 ;5.6 :2013/16].
7.5.1.2 Control of production and service provision — Specific requirements	
7.5.1.2.1 Cleanliness of product and contamination control	
	Does the organization establish documented requirements for cleanliness of product if:
	a) Product is cleaned by the organization prior to sterilization and/or its use, or
	b) Product is supplied non-sterile to be subjected to a cleaning process prior to sterilization and/or its use, or
	c) Product is supplied to be used non-sterile and its cleanliness is of significance in use, or
	d) Process agents are to be removed from product during manufacture?
	If product is cleaned in accordance with a) or b) above, the requirements contained in 6.4 a) and 6.4 b) do not apply prior to the cleaning process.

Doc. Reference	Adequate?	Stage I (clauses marked *)	Stage II

	REQUIREMENTS
Brazil	Confirm that a pest control program has been established and where chemicals are used as part of the pestcontrol program, the company must ensure that they do not affect product quality [RDC ANVISA 2013:5.1.3.4/16]. Verify that the manufacturer has established and maintains housekeeping procedures and schedules forproduction areas and warehouses, in conformance with production specifications [RDC ANVISA 2013:5.1.3.1/16].
7.5.1.2.2 Installation activities	
	If appropriate, does the organization establish documented requirements which contain acceptance criteria for installing and verifying the installation of the medical device?
	If the agreed customer requirements allow installation to be performed other than by the organization or its authorized agent, does the organization provide documented requirements for installation and verification?
	Are records of installation and verification performed by the organization or its authorized agent maintained (see 4.2.4)?
7.5.1.2.3 Servicing activities	
	If servicing is a specified requirement, does the organization establish documented procedures, work instructions and reference materials and reference measurement procedures, as necessary, for performing servicing activities and verifying that they meet the specified requirements?
	Are records of servicing activities carried out by the organization maintained (see 4.2.4)?

Doc. Reference	Adequate?	Stage I (clauses marked *)	Stage II
		*	

	REQUIREMENTS	
Brazil	Confirm that the manufacturer has established and maintains procedures to ensure that records of servicing activities are kept with the following information: the product serviced; the control number of product serviced; the date of completion of service; identification of the service provider; description of service performed; and results of inspections and tests performed [RDC ANVISA :2013/16 8.2.1]. Verify that the manufacturer periodically reviews the records of servicing activities. In cases where the analysis identifies trends that pose danger or records involving death or serious injury, a corrective or preventive action must be initiated [RDC ANVISA 8.2.2 :2013/16].	
7.5.1.3 Particular requirements for sterile medical devices		
	Does the organization maintain records of the process parameters for the sterilization process which was used for each sterilization batch (see 4.2.4)?	
	Are sterilization records traceable to each production batch of medical devices (see 7.5.1.1)?	
7.5.2 Validation of processes for production and service provision		
7.5.2.1 General requirements		
	Does the organization validate any processes for production and service provision where the resulting output cannot be verified by subsequent monitoring or measurement? (this includes any processes where deficiencies become apparent only after the product is in use or the service has been delivered)	
	Does validation demonstrate the ability of the processes to achieve planned results?	

Doc. Reference	Adequate?	Stage I (clauses marked *)	Stage II

	REQUIREMENTS
	Has the organization established arrangements for these processes including, as applicable:
	a) Defined criteria for review and approval of the processes?
	b) Approval of equipment and qualification of personnel?
	c) Use of specific methods and procedures?
	d) Requirements for records (see 4.2.4)?
	e) Re-validation?
	Has the organization established documented procedures for the validation of the application of computer software (and changes to such software and/or its application) for production and service provision that affect the ability of the product to conform to specified requirements?
	Are such software applications validated prior to initial use?
	Are records of validation maintained (see 4.2.4)?
Brazil	Verify that analytical methods, utilities, computer systems and automated software that can adversely affect product quality or the quality system are validated, periodically reviewed and, when necessary, revalidated[RDC ANVISA 5.5.3 ,5.5.2 :2013/16].
Brazil	Verify that processes requiring validation are validated according to previously established protocols. The results of validations, including date and identification of the person responsible for its approval, must be recorded [RDC ANVISA 5.5.1 :2013/16].
7.5.2.2 Particular requirements for sterile medical devices	
	Has the organization established documented procedures for the validation of sterilization processes?
	Are sterilization processes validated prior to initial use?
	Are records of validation of each sterilization process maintained (see 4.2.4)?

Doc. Reference	Adequate?	Stage I (clauses marked *)	Stage II

	REQUIREMENTS
7.5.3 Identification and traceability	
7.5.3.1 Identification	
	Does the organization identify the product by suitable means throughout product realization and does the organization establish documented procedures for such product identification?
	Has the organization established documented procedures to ensure that medical devices returned to the organization are identified and distinguished from conforming product [see 6.4 d)]?
7.5.3.2 Traceability	
7.5.3.2.1 General	
	Has the organization established documented procedures for traceability?
	Do such procedures define the extent of product traceability and the records required (see 8.3 ,4.2.4 and 8.5)?
	Does the organization control and record the unique identification of the product, where traceability is a requirement (see 4.2.4)?
Brazil	Verify that the manufacturer has established and maintains procedures to ensure integrity and to prevent accidental mixing of labels, instructions, and packaging materials [RDC ANVISA 5.2.2.1 :2013/16]. Confirm that the manufacturer has ensured that labels are designed, printed and, where applicable, applied so that they remain legible and attached to the product during processing, storage, handling and use [RDC ANVISA 5.2.2.2 :2013/16].
US	If a control number is required for traceability, confirm that such control number is on or accompanies the device throughout distribution [21 CFR 820.120(e)].

	Doc. Reference	Adequate?	Stage I (clauses marked *)	Stage II

	REQUIREMENTS
EU	Does the manufacturer have procedures identifying the requirements of labeling and instructions for use as defined in MDD, Annex 1 point 13, and is regulations for CE marking included in these procedures. (MDD 3, Article 17 and Annex 12).
	Are language requirements defined in procedures for the information identified in MDD, Annex 1point 13 for the applicable markets.
7.5.3.2.2 Particular requirements for active implantable medical devices and i	
	In defining the records required for traceability, does the organization include records of all components, materials and work environment conditions, if these could cause the medical device not to satisfy its specified requirements?
	Does the organization require that its agents or distributors maintain records of the distribution of medical devices to allow traceability and that such records be available for inspection?
	Are records of the name and address of the shipping package consignee maintained (see 4.2.4)?
7.5.3.3 Status identification	
	Does the organization identify the product status with respect to monitoring and measurement requirements?
	Is the identification of product status maintained throughout production, storage, installation and servicing of the product to ensure that only product that has passed the required inspections and tests (or released under an authorized concession) is dispatched, used or installed?
7.5.4 Customer property	
	Does the organization exercise care with customer property while it is under the organization's control or being used by the organization?

Doc. Reference	Adequate?	Stage I (clauses marked *)	Stage II
e medical devices			

	REQUIREMENTS
	Does the organization identify, verify, protect and safeguard customer property provided for use or incorporation into the product?
	If any customer property is lost, damaged, or otherwise found to be unsuitable for use, is this reported to the customer and are records maintained (see 4.2.4)?
7.5.5 Preservation of product	
	Has the organization established documented procedures or documented work instructions for preserving the conformity of product during internal processing and delivery to the intended destination?
	Does this preservation include identification, handling, packaging, storage and protection, and also apply to the constituent parts of a product?
	Has the organization established documented procedures or documented work instructions for the control of product with a limited shelf-life or requiring special storage conditions?
	Are such special storage conditions controlled and recorded (see 4.2.4)?
Brazil	Verify that the manufacturer has established procedures for the packaging of products in order to protect the product from deterioration, damage, or contamination during processing, storage, handling, and distribution [RDC ANVISA 5.2.1 :2013/16].
7.6 Control of monitoring and measuring devices	
	Does the organization determine monitoring and measuring to be undertaken and the monitoring and measuring devices needed to provide evidence of conformity of product to determined requirements (guide reference 7.2.1)?

	Doc. Reference	Adequate?	Stage I (clauses marked *)	Stage II

	REQUIREMENTS	
	Has the organization established documented procedures to ensure that monitoring and measurement can be carried out and are carried out in a manner that is consistent with the monitoring and measurement requirements?	
	Where necessary to ensure valid results, is measuring equipment:	
	a) Calibrated or verified at specified intervals, or prior to use, against measurement standards traceable to international or national measurement standards; where no such standards exist, is the basis used for calibration or verification recorded?	
	b) Adjusted or re-adjusted as necessary?	
	c) Identified to enable the calibration status to be determined?	
	d) Safeguarded from adjustments that would invalidate the measurement result?	
	e) Protected from damage and deterioration during handling, maintenance and storage?	
	Does the organization assess and record the validity of the previous measuring results when the equipment is found not to conform to requirements?	
	Does the organization take appropriate action on the equipment and any product affected?	
	Are records of the results of calibration and verification maintained (see 4.2.4)?	
	When used in the monitoring and measurement of specified requirements, is the ability of computer software to satisfy the intended application confirmed prior to initial use and reconfirmed as necessary ?	

Doc. Reference	Adequate?	Stage I (clauses marked *)	Stage II

	REQUIREMENTS	
8 Measurement, analysis and improvement		
8.1 General		
	Does the organization plan and implement the monitoring, measurement, analysis and improvement processes needed:	
	a) To demonstrate conformity of the product?	
	b) To ensure conformity of the quality management system?	
	c) To maintain the effectiveness of the quality management system?	
	Does this include determination of applicable methods, including statistical techniques, and the extent of their use?	
Brazil	Verify that the organization has established and maintained procedures for identifying valid statistical techniques required for verifying the quality system performance and process capability for achieving established specifications [RDC ANVISA 9.1 :2013/16].	
8.2 Monitoring and measurement		
8.2.1 Feedback		
	As one of the measurements of the performance of the quality management system, does the organization monitor information relating to whether the organization has met customer requirements?	
	Have the methods for obtaining and using this information been determined?	
	Has the organization established a documented procedure for a feedback system [see 7.2.3 c)] to provide early warning of quality problems and for input into the corrective and preventive action processes (see 8.5.2 and 8.5.3)?	
	If national or regional regulations require the organization to gain experience from the post-production phase, does the review of this experience form part of the feedback system (see 8.5.1)?	

Doc. Reference	Adequate?	Stage I (clauses marked *)	Stage II

	REQUIREMENTS
Brazil	Verify that each manufacturer has established and maintains procedures to receive, examine, evaluate, investigate and document complaints. Such procedures must ensure that: (1) Complaints are received, documented, analyzed, evaluated, investigated and documented by a formally designated unit; (2) Where applicable, complaints must be reported to the competent health authority; (3) Complaints must be examined to determine whether an investigation is necessary. When an investigation is not done, the unit must maintain a record that includes the reason that the investigation was not performed and the name of the responsible for that decision; (4) Each manufacturer must examine, evaluate and investigate all complaints involving possible nonconformities of the product. Any claim for death, injury or threat to public health must be immediately reviewed, evaluated and investigated. (5) The records of the investigation must include: Product name; Date of receipt of the complaint; Any control number used; Name, address and telephone number of the complainant; Nature of complaint; and Data and research results including actions taken [RDC ANVISA 7.2 :2013/16].
8.2.2 Internal audit	

Doc. Reference	Adequate?	Stage I (clauses marked *)	Stage II

	REQUIREMENTS	
	Does the organization conduct internal audits at planned intervals to determine whether the quality management system	
	a) Conforms to the planned arrangements (see 7.1), to the requirements of this International Standard and to the quality management system requirements established by the organization?	
	b) Is effectively implemented and maintained?	
	Is an audit programme planned, taking into consideration the status and importance of the processes and areas to be audited, as well as the results of previous audits?	
	Are the audit criteria, scope, frequency and methods defined?	
	Does selection of auditors and conduct of audits ensure objectivity and impartiality of the audit process (e.g. auditors shall not audit their own work)?	
	Are the responsibilities and requirements for planning and conducting audits, and for reporting results and maintaining records (see 4.2.4) defined in a documented procedure?	
	Does management responsible for the area being audited ensure that actions are taken without undue delay to eliminate detected nonconformities and their causes?	
	Do follow-up activities include the verification of the actions taken and the reporting of verification results? (see 8.5.2)	
Brazil	Verify that quality audits are conducted by trained people in accordance with established audit procedures [RDC ANVISA 7.3.2 :2013/16].	
8.2.3 Measurement and monitoring of processes		
	Does the organization apply suitable methods for monitoring and, where applicable, measurement of the quality management system processes?	

Doc. Reference	Adequate?	Stage I (clauses marked *)	Stage II

	REQUIREMENTS
	Do these methods demonstrate the ability of the processes to achieve planned results?
	When planned results are not achieved, is correction and corrective action taken, as appropriate, to ensure conformity of the product?
Brazil	Verify that processes which cannot be fully verified are conducted in accordance with established procedures and parameters to ensure conformance to specifications. Critical parameters should be monitored and recorded in the batch record [RDC ANVISA 5.1.6 :2013/16].
8.2.4 Monitoring and measurement of product	
8.2.4.1 General requirements	
	Does the organization monitor and measure the characteristics of the product to verify that product requirements have been met?
	Is this carried out at appropriate stages of the product realization process in accordance with the planned arrangements (see 7.1) and documented procedures (see 7.5.1.1)?
	Is evidence of conformity with the acceptance criteria maintained?
	Do records indicate the person(s) authorizing release of the product (see 4.2.4)?
	Does the organization ensure that product release and service delivery do not proceed until the planned arrangements (see 7.1) have been satisfactorily completed?

Doc. Reference	Adequate?	Stage I (clauses marked *)	Stage II

	REQUIREMENTS
Brazil	Verify that the device history record of the product includes or refers to the following information: date of manufacture; components used; quantity manufactured; results of inspections and tests; parameters of special processes; quantity released for distribution; labeling; identification of the serial number or batch of production; and final release of the product [RDC ANVISA 3.2.1 :2013/16]. Verify that labeling has not been released for storage or use until a designated individual has examined the labeling for accuracy. The approval, including date, name, and physical or electronic signature of the person responsible, must be documented in the device history record [RDC ANVISA 5.2.2.3 :2013/16].
Brazil	Verify that sampling plans are defined and based on valid statistical rationale. Each manufacturer must establish and maintain procedures to ensure that sampling methods are suitable for their intended use and are reviewed regularly. A review of sampling plans should consider the occurrence of nonconforming product, quality audit reports, complaints and other indicators [RDC ANVISA 9.2 :2013/16].
8.2.4.2 Particular requirement for active implantable medical devices and im	
	Does the organization record (see 4.2.4) the identity of personnel performing any inspection or testing?
8.3 Control of nonconforming product	
	Does the organization ensure that product which does not conform to product requirements is identified and controlled to prevent its unintended use or delivery?
	Are the controls and related responsibilities and authorities for dealing with nonconforming product defined in a documented procedure?

Doc. Reference	Adequate?	Stage I (clauses marked *)	Stage II
medical devices			

	REQUIREMENTS
	Does the organization deal with nonconforming product by one or more of the following ways?
	a) By taking action to eliminate the detected nonconformity
	b) By authorizing its use, release or acceptance under concession
	c) By taking action to preclude its original intended use or application
	Does the organization ensure that nonconforming product is accepted by concession only if regulatory requirements are met?
	Are records of the identity of the person(s) authorizing the concession maintained (see 4.2.4)?
	Are records of the nature of nonconformities and any subsequent actions taken, including concessions obtained maintained (see 4.2.4)?
	When nonconforming product is corrected, is it subject to re-verification to demonstrate conformity to the requirements?
	When nonconforming product is detected after delivery or use has started, does the organization take action appropriate to the effects, or potential effects, of the nonconformity?
	If product needs to be reworked (one or more times), does the organization document the rework process in a work instruction that has undergone the same authorization and approval procedure as the original work instruction?
	Prior to authorization and approval of the work instruction, is a determination of any adverse effect of the rework upon product made and documented (see 4.2.3 and 7.5.1)?

Doc. Reference	Adequate?	Stage I (clauses marked *)	Stage II

	REQUIREMENTS	
Brazil	Confirm that the evaluation of non-conforming product includes a determination of the need for an investigation and notification of the persons or organizations responsible for the nonconformance. The evaluation and any investigation must be documented [RDC ANVISA 6.5.1 :2013/16].	
Brazil	Verify that the manufacturer has procedures to determine the product recall and other field actions that are relevant in the case of products already distributed [RDC ANVISA 7.1.1.8 :2013/16].	
8.4 Analysis of data		
	Does the organization establish documented procedures to determine, collect and analyse appropriate data to demonstrate the suitability and effectiveness of the quality management system and to evaluate if improvement of the effectiveness of the quality management system can be made?	
	Does this include data generated as a result of monitoring and measurement and from other relevant sources?	
	Does the analysis of data provide information relating to:	
	a) Feedback (see 8.2.1)?	
	b) Conformity to product requirements? (See 7.2.1)	
	c) Characteristics and trends of processes and products including opportunities for preventive action?	
	d) Suppliers?	
	Are records of the results of the analysis of data maintained (see 4.2.4)?	
8.5 Improvement		
8.5.1 General		

Doc. Reference	Adequate?	Stage I (clauses marked *)	Stage II

	REQUIREMENTS
	Does the organization identify and implement any changes necessary to ensure and maintain the continued suitability and effectiveness of the quality management system through the use of the quality policy, quality objectives, audit results, analysis of data, corrective and preventive actions and management review?
	Does the organization establish documented procedures for the issue and implementation of advisory notices and are these procedures capable of being implemented at any time?
Brazil	Verify that procedures and work flows were established in order to identify when field actions (recalls and corrections) are necessary, in accordance with the organization's post-market surveillance system and quality system. [RDC ANVISA 2009/67 RDC ANVISA 2012/23 RDC ANVISA 7.1.1.8 :2013/16]
EU	Are the procedures for Vigilance reporting in conformance with MDD Annex II, V, and VI (MEDDEV 1-2.12)
	Are records of all customer complaint investigations maintained (see 4.2.4)?
	If investigation determines that the activities outside the organization contributed to the customer complaint, is relevant information exchanged between the organizations involved (see 4.1)?
	If any customer complaint is not followed by corrective and/or preventive action, is the reason authorized (see 5.5.1) and recorded (see 4.2.4)?

Doc. Reference	Adequate?	Stage I (clauses marked *)	Stage II

	REQUIREMENTS	
Brazil	Verify that the manufacturer has ensured that information about quality problems or nonconforming products are properly disseminated to those directly involved in the maintenance of product quality and to prevent occurrence of such problems [RDC ANVISA 7.1.1.6 :2013/16].	
	If national or regional regulations require notification of adverse events that meet specific reporting criteria, does the organization establish documented procedures to such notification to regulatory authorities?	
Brazil	Verify that a post-market surveillance system is established and implemented in the organization and integrated into the Quality System, with procedures and work flows established to ensure the correct and the prompt identification of adverse events, the performance of investigations and use of the results to improve the safety and effectiveness of the device when necessary [RDC ANVISA 2009/67 RDC ANVISA 7.1.1.7 :2013/16]	
EU	Are procedures for the reporting of recall to the relevant competent authority and the NB compliant? (MDD, Annex II, V, VI, 3.1)	
8.5.2 Corrective action		
	Does the organization take action to eliminate the cause of nonconformities in order to prevent recurrence and are corrective actions appropriate to the effects of the nonconformities encountered?	

Doc. Reference	Adequate?	Stage I (clauses marked *)	Stage II

	REQUIREMENTS	
	Has a documented procedure been established to define requirements for:	
	a) Reviewing nonconformities (including customer complaints)?	
	b) Determining the causes of nonconformities?	
	c) Evaluating the need for action to ensure that nonconformities do no recur?	
	d) Determining and implementing action needed, including, if appropriate, updating documentation (see 4.2)?	
	e) Recording of the results of any investigation and of action taken (see 4.2.4)?	
	f) Reviewing the corrective action taken and its effectiveness?	
8.5.3 Preventive action		
	Does the organization determine action to eliminate the causes of potential nonconformities in order to prevent their occurrence and are preventive actions appropriate to the effects of the potential problems?	
	Has a documented procedure been established to define requirements for:	
	a) Determining potential nonconformities and their causes?	
	b) Evaluating the need for action to prevent occurrence of nonconformities?	
	c) Determining and implementing action needed?	
	d) Recording of the results of any investigations and of action taken (see 4.2.4)?	
	e) Reviewing preventive action taken and its effectiveness?	

Doc. Reference	Adequate?	Stage I (clauses marked *)	Stage II

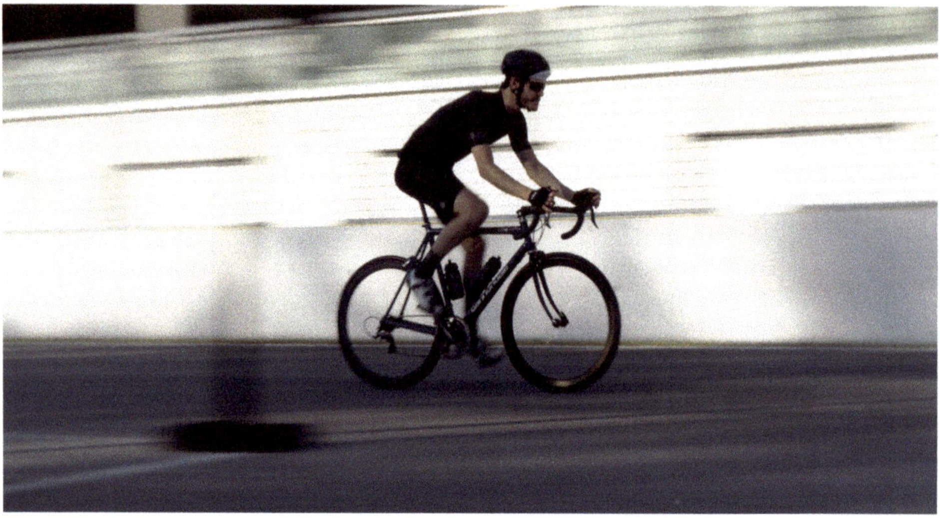

The system is working for you (the system is fully integrated along your processes and eases your operations).

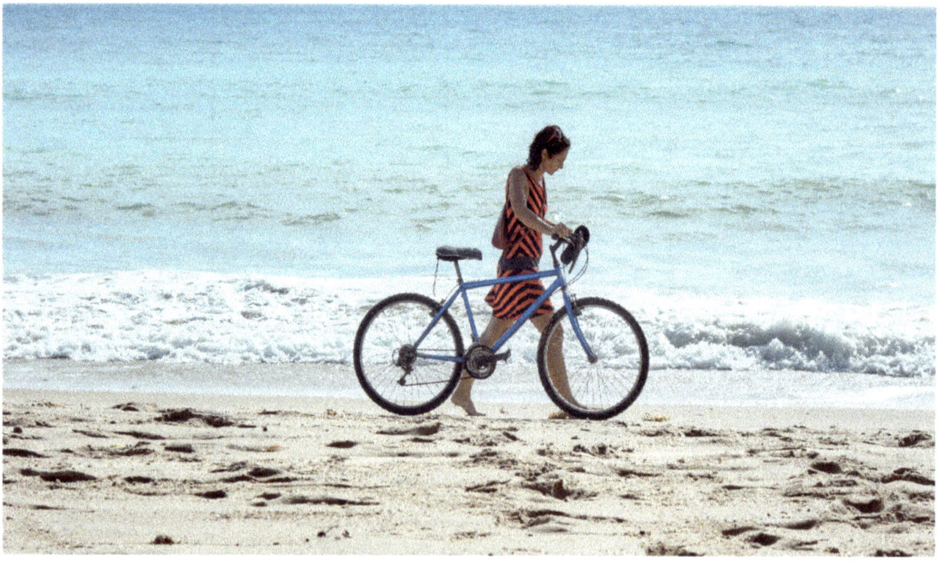

You are working for the system
(the system is beside your operations and looks as an additional burden.)

Advice for manufacturers planning certification

Firstly, you should confirm that the device(s) your company manufactures can be defined as a medical device under ISO 13485 standards; or, if you provide a medical device service, that your service is related to a product defined as a medical device. Getting ISO 13485 certification is challenging and requires commitment so, secondly, it's important that your leadership team confirms that holding the certification will add value to your company, meet its business objectives and support its strategy. While holding the full certification is not strictly necessary, as your company can still conform to and benefit from ISO 13485 standards without being externally certified, it does clearly demonstrate to all stakeholders that you comply with its requirements.

If you do want to become independently certified there are two phases; the first covers documentation, while the second implements your quality management system and audits it. You must carry out phase two within six months of completing phase one.

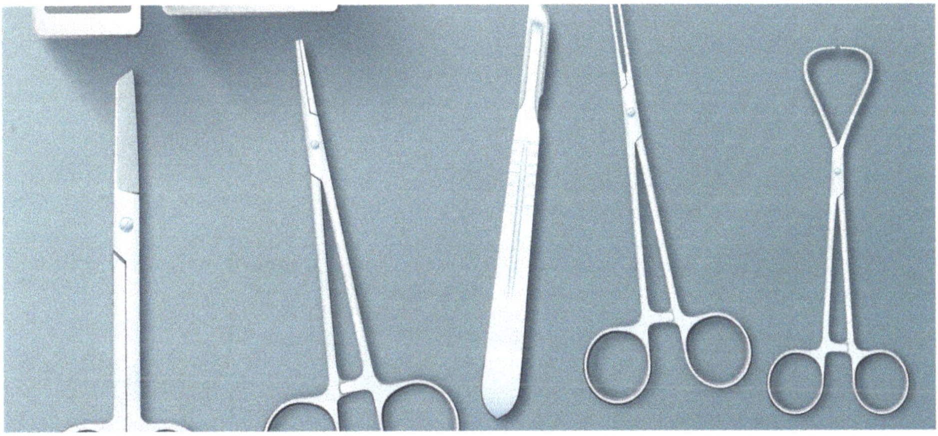

ISO 13485 certification costs

For companies who wish to be fully ISO 13485 certified, there are associated costs for external, independent certification. Although you may be under cost pressure, it's important to work with an independent auditor who will add real value to your company during the certification process. In this highly regulated industry, choose a reputable auditing company with extensive expertise rather than one that enables you to gain certification at the lowest price.

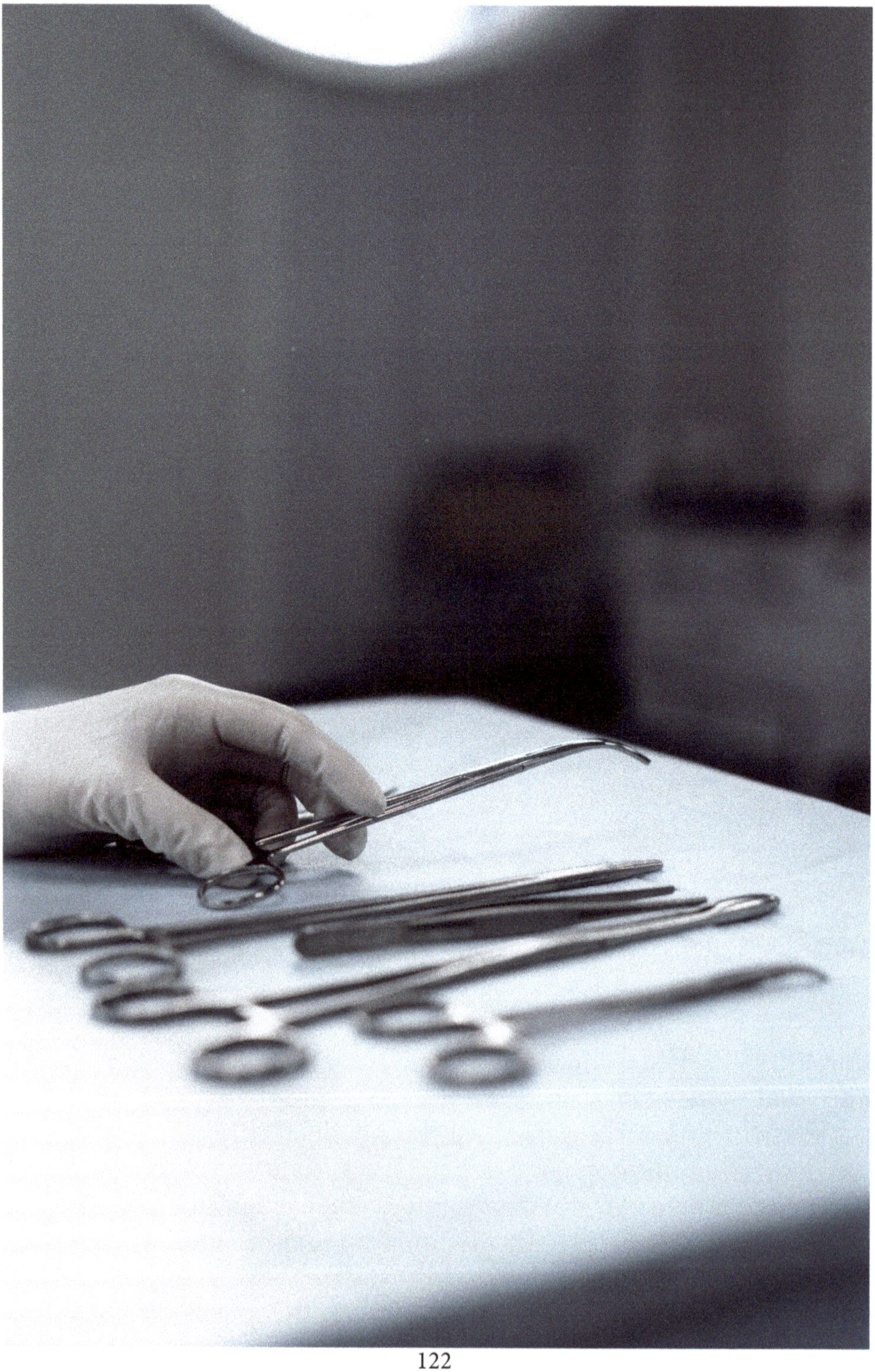

Bibliography

Bibliography:

Astrini, N. (2018). ISO 9001 and performance: a method review. Total Quality Management & Business Excellence, doi: 10.1080/14783363.2018.1524293.

Asadi,J, Easy ISo 13485:2016, Silosa Consulting Group, 2022

Bou-Llusar, J. C., Escrig-Tena, A. B., Roca-Puig, V., & Beltra´n-Martı´n, I. (2005). To what extent do enablers explain results in the EFQM excellence model? International Journal of Quality & Reliability Management, 22(44), 337-353.

Chatzoglou, P., Chatzoudes, D., & Kipraios, N. (2015). The impact of ISO 9000 certification on firms' financial performance. International Journal of Operations and Production Management, 35(1), 145-174. https://doi.org/10.1108/IJOPM-07-2012-0387

Definition of the terms "medical device" and "in vitro diagnostic (IVD) medical device". Global Harmonization Task Force;

Guidelines for regulatory auditing of quality systems of medical device manufacturers – Part 1: general requirements

Global Medical Devices Nomenclature System (GMDN) [website] (https://www. gmdnagency.org, accessed 2 February 2017).

FDA website address: fda.gov

Gigante, N., & Ziantoni, S. (2015). L'edizione 2015 della norma ISO 9001, 2015. Retrieved from:https://www.accredia.it/app/uploads/2015/12/6050_5_L__700_edizione_2015_della_norma_ISO_9001___Arch__Gigante__Dr__Ziantoni.pdf

ISO (2015a). ISO 9001 - Quality management systems – requirements. Geneva: International Organization for Standardization.

Role of standards in the assessment of medical devices. Global Harmonization Task Force; 2008 ISO (2018). ISO 19011 - Guidelines for auditing management systems quality management systems. Geneva: International Organization for Standardization.

ISO (2019). ISO 9000 Family - Quality Management. Retrieved from: https://www.iso.org/home.html.

Wilson, J. P., & Campbell, L. (2018). ISO 9001:2015: the evolution and convergence of quality management and knowledge management for competitive advantage. Total Quality Management and Business Excellence, pp. 1-16. https://doi.org/10.1080/ 14783363.2018.1445965

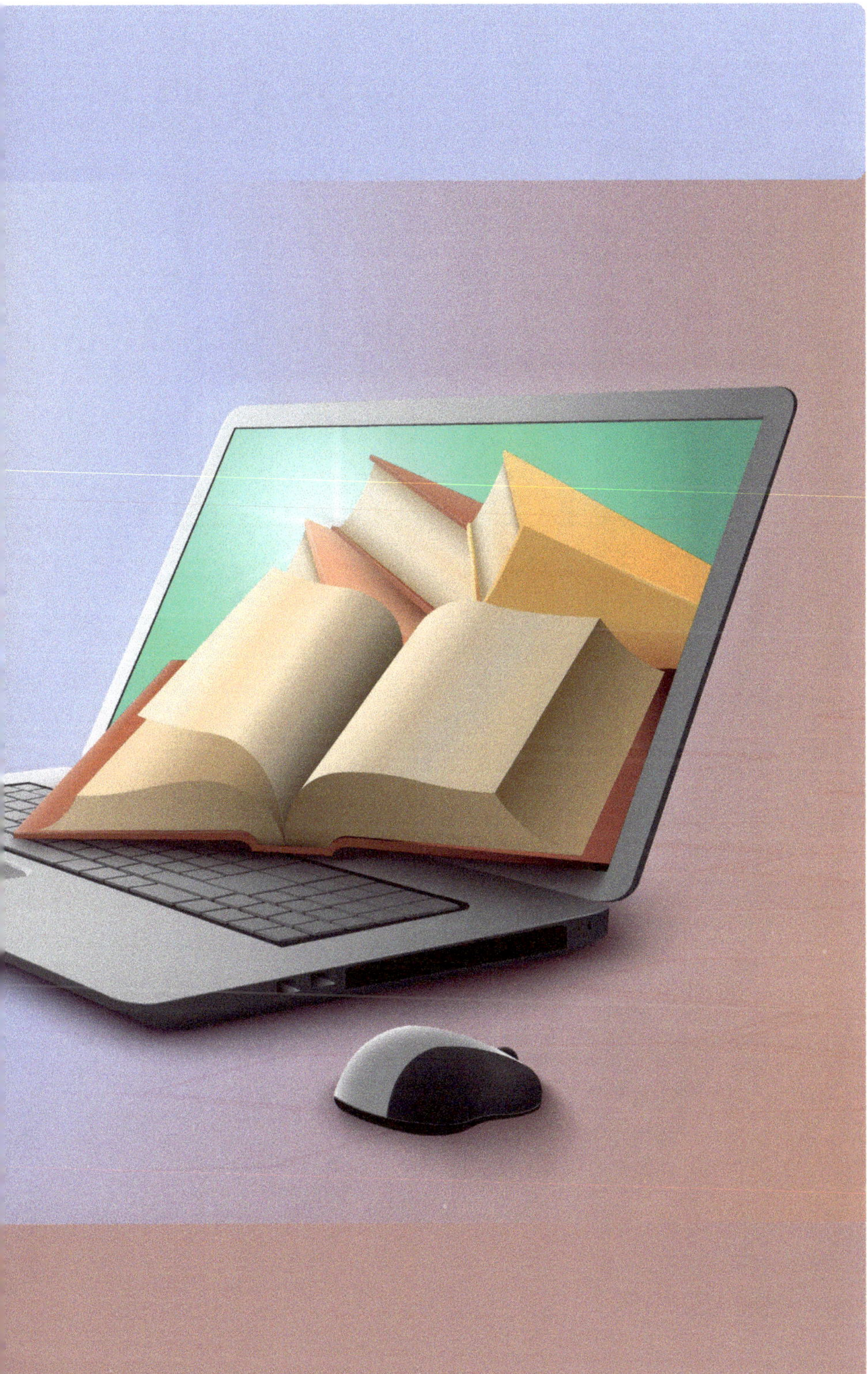

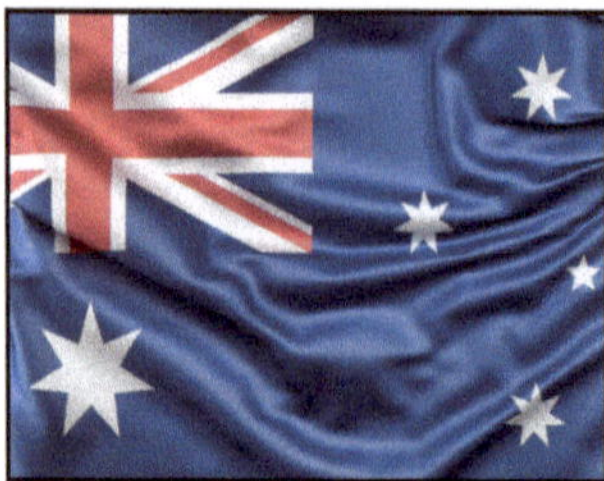

MDSAP

Vol.1

AUSTRALIA

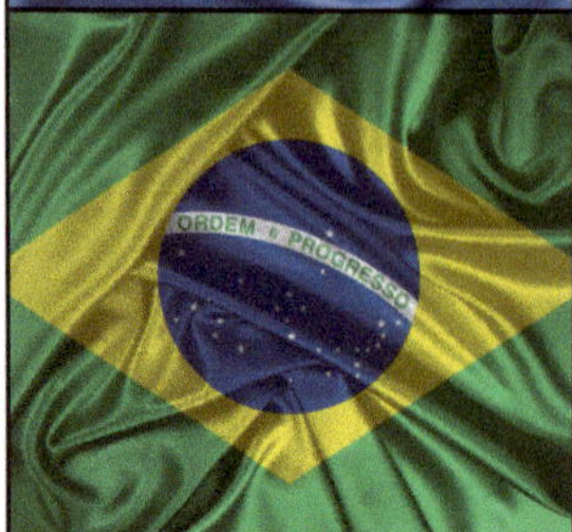

MDSAP

Vol.2

Brazil

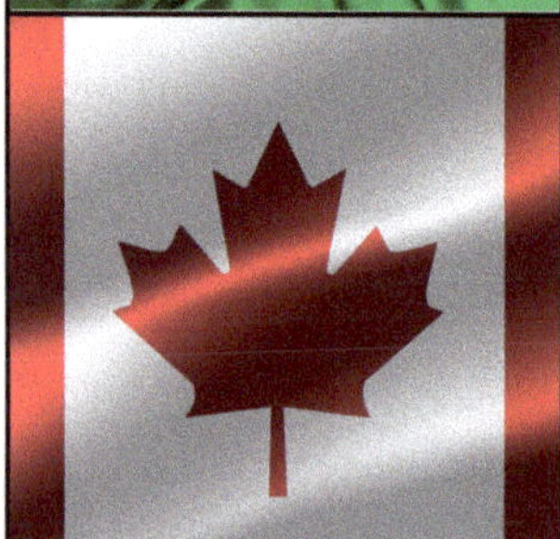

MDSAP

Vol.3

Canada

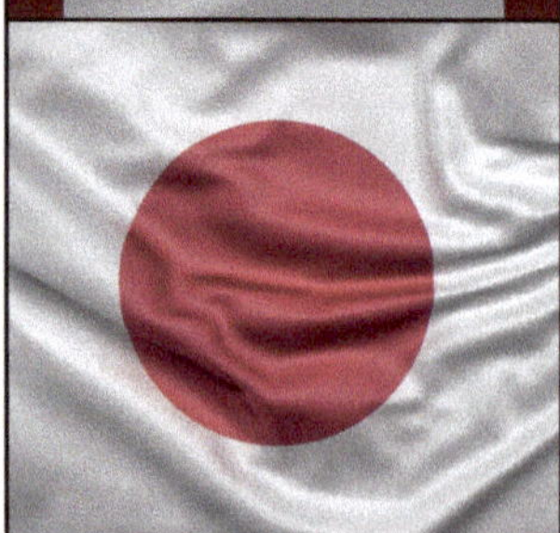

MDSAP

Vol.4

Japan

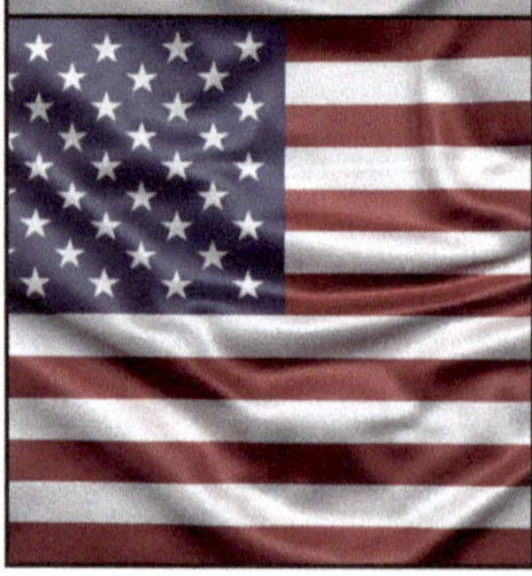

MDSAP

Vol.5

USA

www.ingramcontent.com/pod-product-compliance
Lightning Source LLC
LaVergne TN
LVHW051045210926
848486LV00001B/24

* 9 7 8 1 9 9 0 4 5 1 6 1 4 *